The Complete Guide to Juicing

JUICING

for Weight Loss, Health and Life

Includes The Juicing Equipment Guide

and

97 Delicious Recipes

John Chatham

ROCKRIDGE UNIVERSITY PRESS

ISBNs: Print 978-1-62315-042-6 | eBook 978-1-62315-043-3

TABLE OF CONTENTS

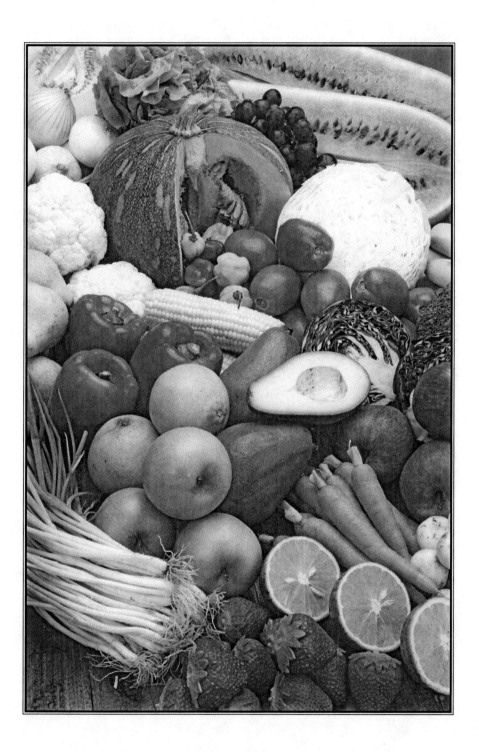

INTRODUCTION

There's a huge trend in the dieting and fitness world right now called juice fasting, but here's a little secret: It's not a trend. People all over the world have been using juices to cleanse the body, prevent illness, and cure diseases for centuries, but it's just now becoming mainstream. So what is it, and how can you do it properly? Excellent questions, and I'm going to do my best to answer them for you.

What Is Juice Fasting?

Juice fasting, also known as "juice cleansing" or just simply "juicing," is exactly what it sounds like: refraining from consuming anything but juice in order to cleanse, detoxify, or heal your body. There are numerous variations of juicing, but all of them involve incorporating the juice from fruits and vegetables into your diet for a set duration of time. In Section 1 of this book, I discuss the technical aspects of juicing, such as the pros and cons, and who can benefit from it.

In juicing's purest form, juice is all that you consume—you don't even drink the pulp. At the other end of the spectrum, many people simply like to incorporate a glass or two of fresh juice, with or without pulp, into their daily diets in order to get a concentrated boost of vitamins and nutrients. Many people also like to do a juice cleanse in order to jump-start a diet plan. Regardless of why you're interested in juicing, there are certain things that you need to know before you start, so I'm here to help you along your way.

What's the Best Way to Extract the Juice?

In Section 2, I'm going to discuss one of the most important components of juicing—how to extract the juice. This is important because the quality of your juicing experience will be affected by the method that you choose. It's a no-brainer that if the process is difficult, messy, or otherwise unpleasant, you're not likely to want to do it on a daily basis.

I've got you covered, though. I'll take the hassle and confusion out of this part of the process by explaining step-by-step exactly what you should look for in a juicer based upon your juicing needs and present living situation. I discuss details that you'd probably never think of so that you're forewarned and forearmed. The section on choosing the right juicer will have you making delicious, nutritious juices with minimal fuss in no time at all.

Is There a Right Way and a Wrong Way to Juice?

Well, yes and no. Because juicing is a personal choice that you make for your own reasons, there really isn't a wrong way to do it if you're just talking about methods or durations. It is, after all, your body. That being said, there are some general guidelines that you should follow in order to get the most out of your juicing experience.

Simple things, like choosing fresh, organic produce and adding herbs and spices to improve both the flavor and nutritional value of your juices, can make a world of difference. I'll explain the top choices of fruits and vegetables, as well as offer some tips on healthy, great-tasting additives that are not only allowed but encouraged.

There are some steps that you need to take prior to starting your juicing experience, especially if you're planning on a total fast. Right now, your body uses about 30 percent of your daily energy just digesting your food because of the fiber and protein that you consume. When you juice, you're eliminating the hard work so that your body is gaining all of the nutrients without needing to expend energy to get them.

That's a pretty big change, and you may experience some initial side effects as your body adjusts. Don't worry, though—I'm not going to let you go in blind. In Section 3, I'll discuss what you need to do to prepare your body for your fast, as well as review some side effects that you may expect. I'll also clue you in regarding how to choose the best produce, what herbs and spices are the most beneficial, and how to maintain your juice fast on the go. As a bonus, for each fruit, veggie, and herb listed, I have included its top nutrients so that you have a reminder even when you're at the grocery store. That means you can make up your own compatible juice combinations right at the market.

So You're Interested in Juice Cleansing?

Though there are many different reasons to juice, cleansing is at the top of the list. Years of eating processed foods filled with excess fat, sugar, and other garbage that your body can't digest leaves your digestive tract stuffed full of junk. The fact that even the air you breathe and the water you drink is full of toxins doesn't help, either. Juice cleansing gets rid of all the trash and helps your body function optimally again. I'll cover how to safely and effectively conduct your cleanse in Section 4.

How to Use Juicing to Stay Healthy and Cure What Ails You

The nutrients, enzymes, antioxidants, and phytochemicals found in fresh fruits and vegetables are amazingly good for you. Antioxidants fight free radicals that cause everything from wrinkles to cancer, and phytonutrients have been linked to a reduced risk of horrible conditions such as stroke, heart disease, and cancer. These benefits are just the tip of the iceberg, but in Section 5, you'll all learn about these awesome disease fighters.

Also in Section 5, I'll discuss which fruits and vegetables offer the nutrients that you're looking for, then I'll take a closer look at some of the most common ailments and reveal the best approach to avoiding and treating them with juice. Each chapter in this section also includes great recipes that are written with a specific condition in mind, just to make your juicing experience a little easier.

It's a proven fact that many diseases can be avoided, at least to a certain extent, just by taking care of your body and providing it with all the nutrients that it needs. There are no magic overnight fixes, though. Good health isn't a sprint; it's a marathon best ran by making one good decision at a time. The decision to add juicing to your diet may be one of the best you'll ever make, so without further ado, let's get you started!

What Is Juicing?

WHAT IS JUICING?

Though you may not realize it, juicing isn't a modern-day innovation, nor is it the result of high-tech research into what's best for your body. Instead, the drinking of fruit and vegetable juices to promote healing and good health has been around practically since the beginning of time. In fact, there are documents that refer to it back as early 150 BC. That's as old as the Dead Sea Scrolls!

In reality, there are many cultures that don't consume any kind of animal protein at all, and eat only raw fruits and vegetables, so the concept of a juice fast isn't quite as extreme as it may initially seem. It's simply an extension of the idea that fruits and vegetables are amazing for you and can be extremely beneficial when looking for a treatment for illness or a boost for your immune system.

Just as there are many different reasons to juice, there are also many different ways to do it. On one end of the spectrum, there are people who consume only low-sugar vegetable juices for as long as months at a time. On the other end, some people simply add a glass of fresh-squeezed orange juice to their breakfast. Regardless of whether you're a hard-core juicer or simply somebody that enjoys a nice glass of juice now and then, there's a spot for you in the world of juicing.

Did you know? *Adding one glass of fresh juice per day to your diet can boost your antioxidant, vitamin, and mineral consumption by as much as 100 percent. That's right—you can literally double your nutrient consumption with one little glass of juice!*

It's not all sunshine and roses, though. There are some definite pros and cons to juicing, especially if you're planning on doing a total fast. Some are more serious than others, and range from mild to yuck. In the following pages, I'll go over what they are so that you can make an informed decision before you decide which level of juicing best suits your needs.

Though most people don't have to worry about it, there are some who may not be able to participate in juice fasting at all because of certain physical conditions. That is OK, because there are still ways that you can reap the benefits of juice while maintaining your health, and without worrying about aggravating your condition.

Now, let's get to the meat of the matter—what the heck is juicing and what can it do for you?

WHAT EXACTLY IS JUICING?

J uice fasting, otherwise known as "juice cleansing" or just plain "juicing," is when you eliminate everything except for the juice from vegetables and fruits from your diet for a certain amount of time. There are many different reasons why you may choose to do a juice fast, but if it's something that you're considering, then the chances are good that it's because you want to cleanse your digestive tract, kick-start a diet, or boost your immune system in order to fight disease.

How Does Juicing Benefit You?

This is, of course, the most important question, so I'm going to answer it before I go any further. I'll talk first about the benefits of doing a total juice fast. If this is what you're choosing to do, then you're not going to be consuming any food at all other than the juice from vegetables, and possibly fruits. The juice is going to be extracted from fresh produce by a special juicing machine, and you're not going to be consuming any pulp at all.

One exception to this juice-only rule is that you are allowed to have certain teas, and you can add certain herbs and spices to your juices and teas as well. As a matter of fact, herbs and spices aren't just allowed, they're actually encouraged because of the health benefits they provide. I'll discuss that in more detail later, though. For now, let's talk about why it's so important to drink only juice and caffeine-free tea while you're fasting.

Easy Access to Nutrients

There's no doubt at all that fiber is good for you, and even essential to a regular diet, but it locks in many of the nutrients that are available in fruits and vegetables. Your body can unlock only a small percentage of the phytonutrients, antioxidants, vitamins, minerals, and enzymes that the fruit or veggie contains. This is because the fiber is really difficult for your body to break down. As a result, most of the good stuff is swept out of your body right along with the waste.

When you're drinking pure extracted juice, all of the nutrients are right there, ready to be absorbed and used. Your body doesn't have to fight to extract them or to use them. You're essentially letting your juicer do the work for your digestive tract so that all your body has to do is absorb all of the good stuff.

Tremendous Energy Boost

Since your body uses about 30 percent of its daily energy supplies digesting food, by eliminating its need to do that work, you're also making a ton of extra nutrients available. Is it any wonder then that you're going to get a boost of energy?

Easy Access to Antioxidants

Antioxidants are amazing little disease-preventing machines that attach themselves to free radicals so that they can't do any additional damage to your body. Free radicals are cells that have become unstable and seek stability by stealing ions from other cells. This causes all kinds of problems, from wrinkles to cancer. Antioxidants are abundant in fruits and vegetables, and are readily available when your body doesn't have to extract them from the fiber.

> **Did you know?** *Your body needs a certain amount of free radicals in order to fight disease and destroy mutated cells. The problem is that they are so good at their job that if they get too abundant, they will destroy healthy cells. Antioxidants are nature's peacekeepers—they make sure that the balance is maintained!*

A Clean Digestive Tract

Your body uses some of the excess energy that it has during a fast to perform some heavy-duty housekeeping. Over the years, you've probably not eaten ideally and have taken in a ton of garbage from processed foods. Your environment is also full of junk, such as toxins and poisons, absorbed by your body on a daily basis. When you're doing a juice cleanse, your body gets rid of all of this trash so that it can function the way that it's supposed to and fight off diseases and illnesses. You'll also actually *feel* lighter as all of the gunk is wiped out.

Improved Cognitive Function

Because you're taking in so many quality nutrients without the added simple sugars, fats, and other junk, in addition to giving built-up toxins the boot, you're going to experience some real cognitive power. It's sort of like an adrenaline shot for your brain—pure, unpolluted energy. All of the nutrients in the juice are going to give your mood a boost, too.

The benefits of participating in a juice cleanse are numerous. You'll feel better, look better, and think better. Your body will be cleaner inside and better able to fight off illness and disease: the flood of nutrients and antioxidants will give your immune system a major kick start. Finally, at the end of your cleanse, your digestive system will work better because it'll be free of years of accumulated garbage.

(2)

THE MANY FACES OF JUICING

There are many different ways to add juice to your diet, and which method you choose depends upon what your goals are. In the following paragraphs, I'm going to discuss how you can add delicious fresh juice to your diet in a manner that best suits your needs and lifestyle. Don't worry—there's something for everybody, so just keep reading until you find what works for you.

Juice Fasting

This is the most extreme way to add juice to your diet, and involves consuming nothing but fresh raw juices, herbal teas, and water for a predetermined amount of time. The purpose of a pure juice fast is to cleanse your body, boost your immune system, and promote healing and good health.

There are a couple of different ways to do this, but the two primary ones are incorporating one day of juice fasting into your diet regularly, or participating in several days, weeks, or months of fasting at a time. There really isn't a right way or a wrong way, as long as you're getting all of the nutrients that you need to stay healthy.

Short-Term Fasting with Both Fruit and Vegetable Juices

This is the easiest and most common way to juice fast, and involves using both fruit and vegetable juices, usually for a period of three to ten days. If you hear the term "juice cleanse," this is what people are referring to. Fruit juices are rich in vitamins and antioxidants but also contain much more sugar than vegetable juice does. As a result, some people report feeling shaky from the sugar rush that they get when they drink fruit juice.

Remember, there's no fiber to slow down absorption, so the sugars in the juice are basically being converted and used for energy immediately. To combat the shaky feeling caused by the instant rush, you may want to limit fruit juice to breakfast, when you need the extra burst of energy, and then use little or no fruit in your recipes for the rest of the day.

Because any kind of a fast can be a shock to your system, there are some steps that you should take in advance in order to prepare your body so that you get the most from your cleanse without getting ill. There are also some side effects that are common with fasting that you need to know about. I'll review the proper way to fast as well as what you can expect in Section 3.

Other Types of Juicing

There are other, more extreme types of juice fasting. Some people limit their fasts to vegetables only. If you choose to do this, make sure that you are getting all of the nutrients that your body needs. Some people also choose to fast for longer periods. As a matter of fact, some people juice fast for months at a time.

Though depriving yourself of any of the major food groups isn't recommended by most doctors or nutritionists, it's your body and thus your choice. If you choose to fast for an extended period of time, make sure that you're getting all of the nutrients that you need to stay healthy.

Be sure to speak with your health-care professional before you start any juice cleanse just to make sure that you're healthy enough to do it.

Simply Adding Juice to Your Diet

This is a method utilized by millions of people every day, and it simply involves adding a glass or two of fresh, raw juice to your daily diet. Whether you drink a glass of fresh orange juice in the morning or prepare something more complicated as a complement to lunch, adding a glass of juice to your diet is an efficient way to get a real nutritional boost.

> **Did you know?** *Millions of people enjoy a glass of fresh orange juice for breakfast, which is great, but the same amount of blueberry juice offers 25 percent of your daily vitamin C, as well as the cancer- and disease-fighting mega-antioxidant anthocyanin. In addition, blueberry juice offers the same protection to your urinary tract that cranberry juice does. Plus, it's delicious!*

Because you're drinking the juice, you're still getting many of the benefits of a fast without actually depriving yourself of solid food. You aren't getting the cleansing properties because you're still eating fiber, but you are getting the antioxidants, vitamins, phytonutrients, and enzymes that your body needs.

Just as there are different levels of fasting, there are also different ways that you can add fresh juice to your daily diet without the deprivation that accompanies a fast. I'll talk about ways to simply add some juice to a healthy, balanced diet in a bit, but first, let's discuss the pros and cons of doing an all-out juice fast.

3

THE PROS AND CONS OF JUICING

Juicing, or any type of fasting for that matter, is tough. Though there are many benefits, there are also some pretty significant downsides. Before starting your juice cleanse, you need to look at it from every angle and decide if you're really ready to see it through, which means discussing the pros and cons of what you're about to do.

Pros

Let's talk first about the benefits that come with a good juice fast. These are based on a fast of three to ten days that includes juice from both fruits and vegetables. Fasting for less than three days is pointless, for a couple of different reasons, while fasting for longer than seven days can actually be detrimental to your health. It's a personal choice, but if you're considering fasting for longer than one week, educate yourself and speak with a nutritionist or health-care professional before making that decision.

Huge Nutritional Boost

When you consume only the juice, you're making it really easy for your body to use the nutrients that are inherent to the juice. There's no digestion, so your body is flooded with just the good stuff, quickly and efficiently. The main components include vitamins, phytonutrients, and antioxidants. It's largely because of this influx of easy-to-use nutrition that you'll experience a boost in energy and mood.

Did you know? *Phytonutrients are organic components of plants that are believed to promote health and wellness. They're not considered essential to survival, but they are conducive to preventing and possibly curing disease and illness.*

Live Enzymes

Enzymes are live protein molecules found in plants that are responsible for many of the chemical reactions in your body. They stimulate digestion, cell building and repair, absorption of nutrients, and the creation of cellular energy. Without these enzymes, your body simply can't function the way that it needs to. Juicing fresh fruits and vegetables is a great way to capture and help your body make use of these enzymes. When juice is pasteurized, as those sold at the grocery store are, the heat kills many of the living enzymes and damages many of the other nutrients as well. Pasteurization is meant to kill any bad bacteria or other bugs that may be living in your food; unfortunately, it also kills the good bugs. You might not get sick, but you also lose much of the nutritional punch that raw juice has to offer.

Clean Digestive Tract

Years of exposure to toxins and eating processed foods that are packed with preservatives leave your gut filled with garbage. After starting a fast, your body will take at least two days to completely rid itself of solid foods and waste that's been lingering in your system. After you're cleaned out, your body can start really using the break from digestion to rebuild cells, fight disease, and flush the toxins from the rest of your body. Consider a good cleanse sort of like a brisk spring-cleaning. Out with the old and in with the new!

Cons

There are definitely some downsides to a juice cleanse that you need to consider before starting one for the first time. Though there's no doubt that you can benefit from a juice fast if you do it correctly, it's also obviously not for everybody. I'm going to touch on a few things to think about before you make any commitments or spend money on a fast that won't be successful for you.

Deprivation

If you opt to do a total juice cleanse, you're going to be depriving yourself of everything but juice, water, and certain herbal teas. There are both physical and mental adjustments that you'll have to make if you're going to be happy and successful with your fast. Some people don't respond well to the idea that they "can't" have something. If you're one of those people, plan accordingly. You can help a bit with the physical aspect of fasting by making sure that you're drinking enough to get all the nutrients that you need as well as taking care to achieve a feeling of fullness that will help keep you sated.

Convenience

Juicing takes some preparation and preplanning, because you're going to have to buy produce, make juice, clean your juicer at least a few times per day, and pack juice to take with you when you go to work or leave the house for any other reason. You'll also probably want to plan so that business or personal meetings don't involve meals; otherwise you're going to be the one person at the table not eating, which could be awkward.

Side Effects

There are certainly side effects to juice fasting. Your body is detoxifying, and you're also switching from a diet that consists of solid foods, fiber, and protein to a diet that is purely liquid nutrients. That's quite an adjustment for your body to make, so you need to be prepared. Some of the side effects are potentially offensive or embarrassing, such as body odor, acne, and bad breath, so if you can, you may want to take a few days off from work and avoid social events.

Taking a few vacation days would be ideal in any case, because you'll have a chance to deal with the side effects as well as adapt to making and drinking the juice. It'll be much less inconvenient if you're fasting on your own schedule. I'll get into side effects in more detail in Section 3 so that you learn even more about what to expect.

Do the Negatives Outweigh the Positives?

Now that you're aware of some of the pros and cons of juicing, you're a little more prepared to make an informed decision. Hopefully you now have a pretty fair idea of whether or not an actual fast is right for you. Remember also that there are other less extreme options that offer many of the same benefits of cleansing without nearly as many downsides, so don't give up on the idea of juicing, even if a fast isn't right for you.

In addition to the cons that I've already touched on, there are some people who really shouldn't do a juice fast at all, or should do so only under the watchful eye of a licensed health-care professional. Juice fasting is extreme and requires adaptations by your body that may not be possible or healthy for people with certain conditions. I'm going to discuss those conditions next.

$$\text{4}$$

TO JUICE OR NOT TO JUICE—
IS IT RIGHT FOR YOU?

Because juicing involves deprivation of fiber and most protein, there are people with certain conditions who shouldn't take on a full-out fast. For the most part, as long as you're healthy and you're not considering fasting for more than a week, fasting should be fine, but read on to make sure that you're in the clear (and consult with your health-care provider when in doubt).

Diabetics

If you have diabetes, you should definitely speak with your health-care professional before starting any juice fast. Your body already has difficulty processing sugar and depends on fiber to slow the process down a bit. When you fast, you're basically absorbing all of the sugar in your juice at once. For somebody with a natural insulin metabolism, that's fine: there will be a bit of an energy burst but no negative health impact. For a diabetic, this sugar spike can be a real issue.

Talk to your doctor about either modifying a juice fast to suit your needs or finding an alternative option that will meet the goals that you wanted to attain via juicing.

> **Did you know?** *If you're diabetic, fresh green vegetable juices can actually help your insulin resistance. If you can't toler-ate the straight juice, try throwing your green veggies into the blender so that you're getting the fiber that you need to slow down the sugar conversion along with the stabilizing effects of the juice.*

Pregnant or Nursing Women

Obviously, if you're pregnant or nursing, you need to talk to your doc-tor about whether or not juice fasting is OK for you and the baby. Your nutritional needs are much different than they are when you're just feeding yourself, and juice fasting is probably not ideal for you right now. For one, you need protein, and so does the baby.

Another thing to remember if you're serious about detoxing is that your body is going to be flushing all of those toxins out in whatever manner it can. Do you really want poisons going into the baby via your blood or breast milk? Finally, your caloric needs are such that, in order to consume enough juice to produce sufficient milk or nutrients for the baby, you'd have to drink almost constantly. It's a better idea to wait until the baby is born and weaned to start a fast or change your diet drastically in any way.

People Who Take Medications

Many medications are dependent upon the digestive process for correct release and distribution. There are also many medications that need to be taken with food in order to prevent nausea or ulcers. In addition to these concerns, juice fasting alters your blood proteins and can affect how your body reacts to your prescription. Because your doctor assumes that you're eating a solid diet with a "normal" caloric intake that includes calories from fiber, fats, and protein as well as beverages, you need to tell him that you're considering juicing when he prescribes a medication. Since some medications are necessary for survival or personal well-being, make sure that you check with your doctor before starting a juice fast.

People with Physical Illnesses or Eating Disorders

When your body is weak from illness, a juice cleanse isn't a good idea. If you've suffered from any kind of eating disorder or other self-image issues, you probably shouldn't start anything as extreme as a fast without consulting your health-care professional to ensure that it's the right decision for you.

Finally, people who have the following ailments or disorders shouldn't participate in a juice fast:

- Cancer
- Epilepsy
- Impaired immune function
- Kidney disease
- Liver disease
- Low blood pressure
- Malnutrition
- Ulcers
- Any other condition that affects your strength or wellness

A better alternative for a detox if you're dealing with any of these conditions is to eliminate processed foods, simple sugars, prepackaged foods, alcohol, and white flour from your diet. Instead, eat organic foods, gluten-free grains, grass-fed proteins, and wild-caught fish; pair these quality meals with fresh juices to reap benefits from both. You'll be eliminating many toxins from your diet just by making these easy changes.

Everything You Need to Know About Juicers

- **Chapter 5:** Juicer, Blender, What's the Difference?

- **Chapter 6:** Types of Juicers

- **Chapter 7:** How to Choose the Perfect Juicer

EVERYTHING YOU NEED TO KNOW ABOUT JUICERS

Choosing a juicer can be confusing, and is quite possibly one of the biggest challenges of your entire juicing experience. If you're new to juicing, you may want to invest in a more economical juicer in the beginning (or borrow one from a friend) until you're sure that you want to stay the course. There are several brands that offer good machines at decent prices, though you may have to sacrifice some of the snazzier convenience features.

In Chapter 5, I'm going to explain what the difference is between a juicer and a blender, and what types of juicers are available. It could be that a simple blender will meet your needs, but if you're serious about participating in a true juice cleanse, then you'll most likely want to go with an actual juicer. Otherwise, you're going to be wasting a lot of time and energy getting what you need from your produce.

Once you've determined whether you need a juicer, there are some points that you're going to want to consider when choosing a machine. Do you know what the difference is between a centrifugal juicer, a masticating juicer, and a triturating juicer? Don't worry—in Chapter 6, I'm going to teach you everything that you need to know to buy your first machine. I'm also going to share some tips so that you can avoid the common first-time buyer mistakes.

Some features are necessary and some are just nice. In Chapter 7, I discuss which features are worth the money. That way, you can decide for yourself whether or not you should spend the extra money.

Finally, I've included a special Juicer Comparison Guide with a handy little list of questions that you can take with you when you go shopping or use to compare features online. Now let's talk juicers!

(5)

JUICER, BLENDER, WHAT'S THE DIFFERENCE?

Excellent question, but once you've read this chapter, you're going to realize that it's an apples-and-oranges comparison. The only real similarity that the two share is that they both produce liquids. That's it. Besides that, the way that blenders and juicers work is totally different, as are the features that each one offers.

Blenders

A blender works by simply grinding up whatever you put into it. It has blades in the bottom of it that rotate at different speeds to achieve the desired consistency. You can make a chunky mixture or a completely smooth one, depending upon how long you blend it, and on what setting.

Even though you can buy different size blenders with anywhere from one to ten speed settings, they all operate in basically the same manner. The ingredients go in the pitcher, the machine gets turned on, the blades revolve, and the contents are broken down and blended.

Juicers

The main purpose (actually, the *only* purpose) of a juicer is to extract the juice from fruits, vegetables, and herbs. Basically, if it grows and has moisture in it, you can put it in a juicer and take out that liquid nutrition. The key is *extracting*, not blending. The major difference between a juicer and a blender is that the end product of a juicer is only juice. No pulp, no skins, no extra "stuff." Just juice.

Did you know? *The first juicer was invented in 1908 by a man named Dr. Norman Walker. It was a centrifugal juicer extremely similar to the ones still in use today. Dr. Walker knew the health benefits of raw juice even then: he lived to the ripe old age of 108!*

Pulp vs. No Pulp

This is actually the crux of the entire blender-versus-juicer debate. Many people prefer to have the fiber that's inherent to the pulp of the produce, but if you're truly juice fasting, then the pulp is a no-no. If you simply want to add some fruits and vegetables to your diet, then the fiber is a great benefit of the produce. It's all a matter of what your goal is.

Now that I've clarified the difference between a blender and a juicer, I need to discuss the different types of juicers. In essence, there are three styles of juicers—masticating, centrifugal, and triturating—and they are distinguished by the way in which they extract the juice from the produce. Which juicer you buy depends on your needs. Consider the following major factors:

- What you're going to be juicing
- How often you'll be juicing
- How much you want to spend

Let's take a closer look at the three juicer types and the terminology and mechanics behind them, and then I'll talk about the importance of key features.

6

TYPES OF JUICERS

All juicers fall into one of the three categories discussed below, though you may also find hybrid machines or ones that are newer versions of the same basic idea.

Masticating Juicers

This type of juicer actually uses an auger or single gear that mashes and chews the produce in order to extract the juice. Masticating juicers tend to operate at low revolutions per minute so they don't produce much heat, which could kill enzymes in the produce. Also, the slow revolutions keep the juice from oxidizing as much, and thus lengthens the shelf life a little.

In addition to making high-quality juices, many masticating juicers also work well to make purees such as baby food, sauces, and nut butters. Many masticating machines extract the majority of the juice from produce and do a good job with difficult leafy vegetables and grasses.

Centrifugal Juicers

The first juicers were centrifugal machines, and though they've advanced in the last several decades with improvements in function and efficiency, they still operate in a similar fashion. Most department store juicers are centrifugal juicers. These machines extract juice in two steps: In the first step, the produce is mashed, and in the second, the pulp is spun so that the juice is pressed out through a strainer. In order to operate at optimal efficiency, these machines must work at higher revolutions per minute (RPM) so more heat is produced. If you're looking for speed, lower cost, and ease of use, this may be the machine style for you.

However, centrifugal juicers tend to extract less juice, and the heat causes oxidation, requiring you to drink the juice immediately. If you're using one of these juicers, you probably won't be able to juice really hard produce, leafy veggies, or grasses efficiently. They are great for soft produce, and fruits without pits and veggies, though. These juicers are also probably the most affordable.

Triturating Juicers

Also known as a "twin-gear juicer," a triturating juicer turns at a slower RPM than other machine types and has a two-step juicing process. In the first step, the produce is crushed, and in the second, it's pressed. This method is excellent for preserving enzymes and getting the maximum nutrients out of produce.

Many triturating machines also make use of advanced technology that slows the oxidation process, helping your juice last longer. Finally, twin-gear juicers are great for juicing dense veggies such as beets and carrots, as well as grasses and leafy produce.

Did you know? *Oxidation begins as soon as the air hits your juice. This is actually the beginning of the spoiling process, and the best way to combat it is to consume your juice immediately. Slow-speed juicers mix less air into the juice, which helps slow the oxidation process.*

Now that you know how the different juicers work, let's take a look at some key features that you'll want to consider when comparing machines.

7

HOW TO CHOOSE THE PERFECT JUICER

Which juicing machine is best for you depends upon several factors. Serious juicers who will be making beet and wheatgrass juice every day and doing a juice cleanse one day a week have vastly different needs than the person who just wants some fresh juice for breakfast. We're going to take a look at the main features that you need to consider when you're trying to find the juicer that's right for you.

First, realize that no juicer is perfect. In order to get some of the features that you want, you may need to sacrifice others, so decide what's most important to you. By doing a little bit of research up front, you'll save yourself time and money later. You'll also avoid buying a juicer that doesn't meet your needs, or has some unexpectedly unpleasant features that may just frustrate you. Now, let's talk juicers!

Key Features

I've drawn from the experience of seasoned juicers to come up with some key features that you want to consider when you're looking at machines. Take these into consideration before you make any decisions.

How Dedicated Are You?

OK, so this isn't exactly a feature of a juicer, but it really is the first thing that you should consider when you're buying one, because they can get pretty pricey. Even cheap juicers run about fifty dollars, and the high-end ones can cost five hundred dollars or more. Since the resale value isn't that great, you may not want to spend big bucks on a machine until you know for sure that you're going to use it more than a few times.

What Are You Going to Juice?

The type of juicer that you buy is largely dependent upon what you need to juice. For instance, if you want to use hard vegetables such as beets and carrots, or would like to use leafy greens and grasses, such as spinach and wheatgrass, you may want to avoid most centrifugal juicers because they don't juice that type of produce as well as triturating or masticating juicers do.

How Noisy Is It?

If you're the first one up and out the door, you might not want a juicer that's going to wake the entire household. If you live alone or are going to make your juice when everybody's up, this may not be as much of an issue. Another factor to consider that goes along with noise is vibration. Some juicers are so light that they'll vibrate right off the counter while you're trying to make your juice. If you can, turn the machine on before buying it. If you can't, read reviews of the product to see what other users have to say about it.

How Long Is the Warranty?

Especially if you're considering spending a significant amount of money on a juicer, you'll want to ensure that your investment is protected by a warranty that covers it for at least one year. Most of the quality machines have one at least that long, and some of them even have limited lifetime warranties.

How Much Heat Does the Juicer Produce?

One of the major benefits of making your own juice is that you get all of the live enzymes and nutrients that are otherwise destroyed during the pasteurization process that store-bought juice undergoes. The main heat source comes from the juicing process itself, specifically the RPM that the machine uses to extract the juice.

Did you know? *Heating juice to more than 118 degrees Fahrenheit kills live enzymes and other beneficial nutrients. Juicers that operate at high speeds often get hotter than those that juice a little slower, so keep this in mind when buying.*

How Easy Is It to Clean?

Because fruits and vegetables are virtual magnets for bacteria that can make you really sick, you must clean your juicer each time you use it. If you're going to be juicing regularly, you especially don't want a machine that takes three hours and a degree in rocket science to take apart and clean. Choose a machine that has as few parts as possible, is dishwasher-safe, and assembles and disassembles easily.

Also, keep in mind that the natural dyes in fruits and veggies will stain plastic. If you're going to keep your juicer on the counter, white might not be the best option.

How Much Space Does It Take Up?

Though juicers that are heavier may be less noisy and won't rattle so much, they're also more difficult to store. If you have plenty of cabinet space, or don't mind the way that the juicer looks sitting on your counter, then this isn't a concern. However, if you don't have much storage space or don't want your juicer sitting out, then you'll want to take the size and appearance of your machine into consideration.

How Big Is the Cup and the Hopper?

This may not seem like such a big deal, but if you need to cut your produce down into smaller pieces in order to juice them, or if the cup holds only a few ounces, then the process may become frustrating and you'll be less likely to stick with your healthy new habit. After all, most people don't have the time or patience to spend two hours making enough juice to get you through the day.

Does It Leak?

This sounds like a no-brainer, but believe it or not, some machines are constructed so poorly that the juice leaks out as it's produced. Check online reviews and inspect the machine closely if you're buying one at the store. The leaked juice is not only a pain to clean up, it's also a waste of your money, time, and effort, and is likely to discourage frequent use.

How Well Does It Juice?

One of the most frustrating things about using a juicer is dealing with the solid waste. If you open up the pulp container and it has as much pulp as it does juice, then you're effectively throwing money down the drain. Typically, a machine needs to have at least one-fourth horsepower (186 watts) in order to properly juice anything. Do some research and pay attention to what other users say about any moisture left in the pulp. Try to go with a juicer that removes as much juice as possible. "Dry pulp" is a key phrase to watch for.

What's Best for You?

Buying a juicer can be confusing, especially if you're new to the process. Many people learn from trial and error, but I've tried to provide you with the most important purchase considerations so that it's as simple as possible. There really is no juicer that's perfect for every scenario, so just do what you can to choose the one that most closely matches your needs.

Below, you'll find a list of questions that you can use to compare the juicers that you're looking at more easily to see which one may be right for you. After that, in Section 3, I'll get into the meat of juicing—what you'll need to do to prepare, how to actually conduct your fast, side effects that you can expect, and what produce is most beneficial.

JUICER COMPARISON GUIDE

Use the following list to compare your top juicer choices. If there are other options that interest you, just fill them into the empty blanks.

	Juicer 1	Juicer 2	Juicer 3	Juicer 4
Name of juicer				
What is the price?				
Will it juice what you need it to?				
How noisy is it? Does it vibrate?				
How powerful is it (horsepower/watts)?				
What kind of warranty does it have?				
How much heat does it produce (RPM)?				
Is it easy to clean?				
How big is the cup and hopper?				
Does it leak?				
How much juice is left in the pulp?				
What color is it?				
How big is it? Will it store well?				

The Healthy Person's Guide to Juicing

THE HEALTHY PERSON'S GUIDE TO JUICING

As you've probably noticed, the title of this section implies that you're healthy. I've already discussed numerous reasons why it's absolutely imperative that you don't juice fast if you're suffering from certain physical conditions, illnesses, or diseases. From this point forward, all tips and advice will be based on the assumption that you're in good health and free of medical issues, because juicing while you're not tip-top can truly do more harm than good. Now that I've got that out of the way, let's get on with juicing!

Preparation Is the Key to Success. Really the title says it all here, but it's the truth. No other single factor can influence the success or failure of your juice fast more than how well you prepare. Because you're going to be consuming no solid foods, toxins, or junk for an extended period of time (at least for a few days), you need to wean your body off these things slowly. Otherwise, you're going to suffer worse side effects and withdrawal symptoms than you need to.

Adding Juice to Your Diet. Because you're going to be taking in only pure, unadulterated nutrition without the fiber to slow down the digestion process, it's a good idea to start adding in some fresh juice to your diet before you go completely off solid food. Just like you're going to wean yourself off everything else, you should be kind enough to your system to let it get familiar with this new form of nutrition that it's going to be surviving on.

Speaking of getting familiar with things, there are other reasons to start adding fresh juice to your diet prior to the morning that you start your cleanse. I'll discuss these in Chapter 9.

Why Use Fresh Juice? This is a question that I'm going to answer in much greater detail in Chapter 10, but the short, sweet answer is that there's really no reason to fast if you're going to use store-bought, bottled juices. The nutrients, live enzymes, and other goodies that are available only in fresh juice are the primary reason that juice fasting is effective. Also, by making your own juices, you can decide what nutrients you're getting and when.

What Are the Best Fruits and Vegetables to Use? It's true that all fruits and vegetables are good for you and provide different nutrients that your body needs. However, when it comes to juicing, all produce is definitely not made the same. For several different reasons, including flavor, nutritional value, and juice ability, there are simply some produce items that stand head and shoulders above others. I'll review the top twenty fruits and the top twenty vegetables so that you know which ones are stellar for juice fasting and why. I'll also touch on a few herbs and spices that will really boost the flavor and nutritional value of your juices.

Side Effects Are Certain. By fasting, you're clearing all of the toxins, heavy metals, and waste from your body. You're also consuming only liquid nutrition, which expedites the digestion process. There are going to be side effects, both good and bad, when you do that. Chapter 15 tells you what you should expect throughout your juice fast, and Chapter 16 offers some tips that will help you get the most out of your juicing experience.

8

PREPARING FOR YOUR CLEANSE

One of the main reasons for considering a juice cleanse is because you want to flush the toxins out of your body, but you probably don't think much about some of the poisons and digestive disablers that you consume on a regular basis. Because juice fasting is an extreme form of dieting, there are several steps that you need to take in order to prepare your body properly and make your cleanse a much more pleasant experience.

Eliminate Drugs

You're in contact with toxins on a daily basis, and some of these you inflict upon yourself. You're an adult who can make that decision, but it's going to make your fast much more difficult. If you choose to smoke, slug down copious amounts of caffeine, or pop in for happy hour on your way home from work, know that ingesting these substances is not conducive to a successful cleanse.

If you're getting ready to juice fast, you don't want to put your body through the traumatic experience of depriving it of those things all at once. Needless to say, your body won't be happy, and you'll suffer for it.

The withdrawal symptoms, including headache, nausea, and moodiness, are going to make you miserable if you quit cold turkey. Your body is going to be dealing with enough changes during your fast, so try to eliminate these particular habits from your life a couple of weeks before you start juicing. Here are the things that you should ditch:

- Alcohol
- Caffeine
- Nicotine
- Over-the-counter medications
- Recreational drugs

If you really want to feel good and be healthy, don't start them again once you've finished your fast, either!

Did you know? *Smoking is as much a psychological addiction as it is a physical one. You're going to be craving that hand-to-mouth habit, so try celery or a carrot stick. It's actually a negative-calorie food, so you won't gain weight.*

Stop Eating Junk

Just like your body can become dependent on drugs, it can also get hooked on many of the unhealthy foods that you eat. It's really easy to just grab something from the freezer section to pop in the microwave for lunch, and a bowl of ice cream while you're watching TV at night is delicious, but neither of them is good for you. Not only are they bad for your body, but they can actually be addicting.

Your body gets used to having the extra sugar, sodium, et cetera, and when you stop eating those foods, you'll go through withdrawal. Since you don't want to stop all of your bad habits at once, wait until a week or so before your fast to start weaning yourself off the following juicing no-no's:

- Artificial sweeteners
- Dairy products
- Fried foods
- Meat
- Processed foods
- Salt
- Sugar
- Sushi
- White flour

Again, if you want to be healthier after your fast, consider leaving the majority of these off your daily menu permanently.

Ditch the Gluten

This one's not really so much an addiction that will make you sick as it is just a habit that you should kick to make your fast a little easier. Since you're not going to be eating any bread for the duration of your fast, it'll be easier for you to wean yourself off it than to just quit eating it all at once. Start eliminating these products three days or so before your fast:

- Bread
- Oatmeal
- Other oat, barley, rye, or wheat products
- Pasta

If you're eating healthy forms of these foods, you can add them back into your diet when your fast is over. Just for general health though, if you're eating white pastas and breads made with refined flour, consider switching to whole grains. They taste better and are much better for you.

Add Raw Foods

If you're a typical person, you'll be eliminating most of your regular foods while you're juice fasting. Even if you eat a relatively healthy diet, you're still probably eating meats, dairy, and wheat products. That means that, when you fast, you're basically hitting the brakes on just about everything your digestive tract is used to.

To prepare your body even more thoroughly for your fast, start adding in raw fruits and vegetables while you're weaning yourself off the other stuff. That way you're not starving while still eating solids, and your body is starting to get used to a modified version of what it's going to be living on during the fast. Add more of the following items to your diet as you eliminate the others:

- Fresh juice
- Leafy green salads and sprouts
- Non-caffeinated herbal tea
- Raw fruits and vegetables
- Vegetable soup
- Water

Prepare Your Mind

Not only do you need to prepare your body for the juice cleanse, you also need to prepare your mind. Any time you make serious changes to your routine, you're adding stress to your life. It doesn't really matter whether or not the change is positive or negative; the stress is still there, and your mind has to adjust to the new way of doing things.

Since you're going to be depriving yourself of many things that you enjoy, as well as toxins that your body may be addicted to, it's important to find a way to relieve the stress and anxiety that inherently accompanies that process. What follows are a few ways to prepare your mind while preparing your body.

Exercise

You're not going to be able to exercise vigorously because it's likely that you'll be a little weak and will have less endurance, but exercising is still a vital part of keeping your mind straight and your body healthy. Especially if you're used to working out on a daily basis, continue exercising even if you have to modify your routine a little.

Meditate

This is a great way to clear your head and relieve stress. There are as many ways to meditate as there are people in the world, but find what works for you and practice it. Even if it's just a matter of sitting quietly and clearing your mind, or listening to your favorite music without focusing on anything in particular, give your mind a break for a few minutes each day.

Concentrate on the Positive

You've decided to start a juice fast for a reason. Whether it's because you want to kick-start a diet, clean out your digestive tract, or clear your body of disease, there's a positive motivation behind the decision. Write down all of your reasons and read them if you start feeling negative or unsure. Surround yourself with people who support you and keep your goals in mind at all times. If you really get the urge for a huge plate of spaghetti or a candy bar, just remind yourself why you decided to fast to begin with and what you have to gain by completing it.

Now that you've got your body and mind prepared for your fast, let's talk about ways to start introducing wonderful fresh juices into your diet.

9

ADDING JUICE TO YOUR DIET

Your body probably isn't used to digesting fresh, pure juice, so just adapting to that change is going to be challenging for your system. You'll do better when you take a break from solid foods if your body (and your palate) is already used to the juice, so starting adding it to your diet even before you begin your fast.

Get to Know Your Juicer

The last thing you want to do is wait until the first day of your juice fast to figure out your juicer. You really don't want to find out twenty minutes before you need to leave for work that your machine won't juice half of the produce that you bought, even though it says that it will on the box. Start playing with it a week or so in advance so that you know it inside and out and can juice your produce and clean the machine comfortably.

Start with Good-Tasting, Familiar Juices

You're not going to stick with your fast if you don't like the taste of your juice. If every meal is a punishment that requires squeezing your nose and gulping, you'll never last through the entire fast. Start playing with flavors while you're learning how to use your machine. That will give you a chance to figure out which flavors appeal to you and which ones don't.

Did you know? *Produce that's completely ripe not only tastes better, it also yields up to twice as much juice and has more nutrients, too. If possible, don't buy your produce more than a couple of days in advance, because many fruits and veggies don't get any more ripe once they're picked. They just rot and you lose the nutritional value and taste.*

The best way to get yourself used to juices is to start out with ones that you know that you like. For instance, most of us have had the most popular fruit juices. Use those as a base and try adding familiar, good-tasting vegetables to them. Here are a few that are pleasant tasting and may work well with your fruit juices:

- Beets
- Carrots
- Celery
- Cucumbers
- Potatoes
- Tomatoes

You're probably already used to the flavor of tomato-based juices (think Bloody Mary!), and you'll be pleasantly surprised at how many great-tasting juices you can make just by building on this base. Especially if you're willing to spice them up with herbs and seasonings, it won't take you long to love tomato-based creations. Get creative—throw some spinach or broccoli into your tomato cocktail, along with some garlic, horseradish, or maybe some cayenne pepper. Start backing down on the tomato and switching to just the greens. Green juice really can taste good once you get past the fact that it's not the most appetizing color!

If you start adding juice into your regular diet as you start eliminating the bad foods, then by the time you are ready to actually start your fast, you'll be a pro. You'll have a good idea of what you like and what you don't, and you'll know how to use your machine. Best of all, you won't be making a sudden, huge change, either physically or mentally. By preparing your body and mind, you're setting yourself up for a successful juice fast.

Now that you know how to get ready for your fast, let's discuss why it's so important that you make your own juice instead of buying it at the store. There really is a world of difference between what you can make at home and what you get from a bottle, and those differences are magnified when it comes to juice fasting. As a matter of fact, if you're going to use juice from a bottle, you may as well skip the fast altogether. That may seem harsh, but let's examine why it's true.

KEEPING IT FRESH—TOP 3 REASONS TO MAKE YOUR OWN JUICE

If you look on the shelves of your local grocery or health-food store, you're going to find dozens of different juices. There's juice with pulp and juice without. You'll find single juices, juice blends, and juice drinks. You'll even find juices that claim to be 100 percent pure, with no additives or preservatives. Are these juices good for you? Some of them definitely are, but not a single one of them is acceptable for a juice fast.

Why not? The main reason is because the vast majority of commercially produced juices are chock-full of much of the nasty stuff that you're trying to rid your body of during your cleanse. Another major reason is that those packaged juices just don't contain the nutrients that fresh juice made at home and consumed immediately does. Let's take a look at the main reasons that you need to make your own juice.

Added Junk

Many of the juices for sale at the store contain added sugar, salt, preservatives, and chemicals. There's no way to really know what's in the bottle, even after reading the ingredients. Unfortunately, there's not even a guarantee of any significant amount of juice in the bottle. Especially in juices with labels that say "juice blends" or "juice drinks," there are often only small percentages of actual juice. The rest of the drink is nothing but artificial flavors, colors, sugar, and preservatives, and that's exactly what you're trying to get *out* of your system!

Added Poison

In addition to all of the icky additives in those juices, you also have to think about the pesticides and other poisons that were present on the fruit when it was grown and processed. There's no guarantee that the fruit was organic, or that it was processed in an environment that was free of contamination. Again, you're trying to flush all of that garbage out of your body, not add more in.

Nutritional Value

Fresh juice still contains all of the delicate live enzymes, vitamins, and nutrients that were present in the fruit itself. Also, the skin of the produce protects the juice from oxidation, which is a chemical reaction that occurs when oxygen hits the enzymes in the produce, turning items such as apples, plums, and potatoes brown. It's actually the destruction of the enzyme that you're watching, and the start of decay. Obviously, this takes away from the nutritional value of the juice!

In addition to oxidation, you also have to remember that most juices are required to undergo pasteurization according to health regulations. This involves the juice being heated to a certain temperature in order to kill pathogenic bacteria (the kind that can make you sick). Manufacturers also use the process to kill the bacteria that cause spoiling so that they can extend shelf life and reduce product waste. Pasteurization not only kills the bad bacteria, it also kills the good enzymes and nutrients, and changes the flavor.

As you can see, it really is necessary to make your own juice at home in order to avoid pesticides, additives, and preservatives. You also get all of the natural nutrition that's present in the fresh produce. There are a few other reasons why homemade juice is better, too:

- Pure taste
- You know for sure what's in it
- You can make your own flavor profiles
- You can create a juice that meets your nutritional goals
- You can make as much or as little as you want

The bottom line is that if you're going to fast correctly, you need to make your own juices for the maximum benefit. By buying your own produce and creating your own combinations, you control exactly what you're putting into your body and, thus, can get the most out of your fast.

Now that you understand why you need to make your own juice, let's talk about the differences between fruit juices and vegetable juices, and the pros and cons of each.

(11)

FRUIT JUICE VS. VEGETABLE JUICE

I f someone were to offer you a glass of orange juice fresh from the press or a glass of broccoli juice, which one would you choose? Probably the orange juice, right? That's because it's a classic fruit juice you've probably been drinking all of your life. It's good for you and it's delicious. But it doesn't provide you with all of the nutrients that you need to survive.

Just as when you're eating solid food, you need to consume a variety of fruits and vegetables when you're juice fasting. In the following paragraphs, I talk about the differences between various fruits and vegetables, and why it's important for you to consume them both.

Fruits

For the sake of this discussion, I'm going to use the culinary standpoint when determining what is a fruit and what is a vegetable: fruits are the sweet stuff, such as oranges, pineapples, cherries, and so on. In other words, I don't care about where the seed is.

Now that I've gotten that straight, the primary difference between fruits and vegetables is the sugar content. Because you'll only be drinking the juice and none of the pulp to slow down digestion, you may want to avoid juicing many fruits by themselves. The sugar will be quickly absorbed and converted to energy, and the resulting burst may cause dizziness, nausea, and possibly a headache.

Use fruit juice sparingly during your cleanse. If possible, try to limit your fruit-only juice intake to breakfast and small snacks. Also, aim to limit the amount of fruit in the rest of your recipes to just one. Don't skip fruits completely, though—they have some amazing nutrients in them! Just be sure to consume fruits in moderation.

Vegetables

Possibly the easiest way to differentiate between the nutritional content of your veggies (and fruits) is by color. If you separate vegetables into purples, greens, and yellows, you'll find that each offers unique nutrients and health benefits. Every yellow vegetable and fruit doesn't offer exactly the same vitamins and minerals, but most of them share some common characteristics. On that note, it's entirely possible that going by color will be easier than trying to remember fruit and veggie classifications, and what nutrients they offer.

Yellows

Yellow and orange produce, such as carrots, squash, citrus fruits, apricots, and sweet potatoes, all contain carotenoids, vitamin C, and lutein. In addition to being excellent for your eyes, these nutrients are also great for fighting cancer and other diseases. A bonus is that the vitamin C will help keep your juices from oxidizing. When you put fresh lemon juice on apple slices, for example, the apples will oxidize much slower than they would otherwise.

Greens

You always hear it—eat your greens. Well, there's a reason for that. Bright green fruits and veggies, such as broccoli, Brussels sprouts, kale, cabbage, spinach, peas, and avocados, are rich in carotenoids, niacin, and vitamins A, C, and B6. Many of them are also packed with minerals such as potassium, calcium, and magnesium. In addition to fighting disease, these nutrients are great for your cardiovascular system, your immune system, and your bones. Drink your greens!

Purples

Red, purple, and blue fruits and veggies, such as blueberries, beets, grapes, cherries, plums, and red cabbage, are rich in the flavonoid anthocyanin, which is a plant pigment and antioxidant that protects cells from damage, fights cancer, and may prevent heart disease and stroke. In addition, many of the purples, blues, and reds also have lycopene, another free-radical fighter that's great for your eyes.

This is just a general guide to help you remember that when you're making your juices, you should try to incorporate a variety of produce in order to get the most from your cleanse. Now that you have a thumbnail guide, let's talk about the top twenty fruits and vegetables. As an aside, many fruits and vegetables are only available in the spring and summer, so this may be the best time to complete your juice cleanse.

Did you know? *Polyphenols, particularly those from blueberries, are being studied for their potential ability to help reduce high blood-glucose levels. This is being looked at closely because of the potential for diabetic and weight-control uses.*

(12)

TOP 20 FRUITS AND
WHY THEY MADE THE LIST

To start, let's just say that this wasn't an easy list to come up with. Every fruit has unique and beneficial nutritional properties, but some are just that much better than others. In addition to nutritional value, I also took into consideration the ease of juicing and the availability of the produce when composing this alphabetical list.

Apples

The old saying "an apple a day keeps the doctor away" has proven time and again to be true. Apples have numerous health benefits, but these are the top three things they do for you:

- **Asthma risk reduction**—Though it's not fully understood why, apples reduce the risk of asthma. Researchers theorize that the antioxidant and anti-inflammatory properties of apples play a role, but it's so pronounced that it can't be attributed to those alone. They are pretty amazing fruit!

- **Blood sugar regularity**—The phytonutrient known as polyphenol is known to help regulate blood sugar; apples are packed with several different kinds.
- **Cancer risk reduction**—Apples are packed with antioxidants and are known to help prevent several different types of cancer, including colon and breast cancers. There's also an unexplained link between apples and a reduced risk of lung cancer. Research in this area continues in order to determine the connection.

> **Did you know?** *Apple juice has been used for centuries as a holistic treatment for liver problems, memory loss, cancer prevention, and constipation.*

Apricots

Beautifully orange and deliciously sweet, apricots are a smaller cousin of peaches. They taste a little bit musky, with a moderately sweet tartness. Apricots have the following benefits:

- **Eye health**—The antioxidants in apricots include vitamins A and C. These vital antioxidants are known to fight the free radicals that cause age-related macular degeneration.
- **Heart health**—The beta-carotene in apricots may contribute to healthy levels of good (HDL) cholesterol, and may help prevent heart disease.

Bananas

Technically, bananas shouldn't be included on this list because you can't juice them, but the health benefits are so significant that they couldn't be left off. Though you can't consume them during a juice fast, you can certainly incorporate them into smoothies outside of your fast or just incorporate them into your regular diet to get a boost.

Packed with vitamins C, K, and B6, bananas also have potassium, magnesium, and manganese. Fun fact: Almost all of the vitamin K in a banana is found in that little tip that many of us cut off and throw away! Bananas help your body in the following ways:

- **Blood pressure maintenance and heart health**—As one of the best sources of potassium on the planet, bananas play a huge role in helping keep your blood pressure regulated so that you can avoid strokes and heart attacks.
- **Bones strength**—Bananas are a rich source of the prebiotic fructooligosaccharide. This nourishes the probiotics in your colon and throughout your digestive tract. Probiotics control bad bacteria and produce digestive enzymes so that your colon can absorb the nutrients that it needs. One of the things that probiotics do is help your colon absorb calcium, which we all know keeps bones strong.
- **Ulcer relief**—Bananas help your stomach in two ways. First, a chemical in them stimulates the mucous cells that line your stomach. Second, the protease inhibitors in bananas actually reduce acid secretion. In studies, a simple mixture of milk and banana significantly reduced acid secretion in the stomach.

Blueberries

These little round powerhouses are incredible for you. As a matter of fact, just a handful of them help you avoid a wide array of illnesses. When you're not juicing, grab a few of these for a snack instead of potato chips if you want to live longer and feel better. They're packed with vitamins K and C, and manganese, and are absolutely bursting with phytonutrients. Here are some of their great benefits:

- **Antioxidant support**—Not only have blueberries been shown to provide antioxidant support to certain bodily systems, they protect your *entire* body. For example, studies are showing that eating blueberries reduces damage to muscles following strenuous exercise. They also protect against neurodegenerative diseases.
- **Brainpower boost**—Studies are showing that adults who drink blueberry juice show improved scores on cognitive tests, including memory and other age-related issues. Research indicates that this may be because the antioxidants protect nerve cells and encourage healthy oxygen metabolism.
- **Blood sugar level maintenance**—Studies following people who have insulin resistance, metabolic syndrome, type 2 diabetes, and obesity indicate that blueberries assist with maintaining healthy blood sugar levels, even in people for whom it's a challenge.
- **Cancer protection**—Because of the superhero level of antioxidants and phytonutrients in blueberries, it's no surprise that they help protect you from cancer of the breast, colon, small intestine, and esophagus. These are just the ones that have been studied, so it won't come as a surprise if other cancers turn up on the list in the future.
- **Cardiovascular defense**—Antioxidant support is particularly potent in the cardiovascular system. Blueberries help lower bad cholesterol, raise good cholesterol, and protect your blood from oxidative damage. Blueberries also increase antioxidant protection in blood and plasma, helping your blood vessels. Finally, blueberries can reduce high blood pressure and help maintain a normal blood pressure.
- **Eye health**—Blueberries reduce the oxidative stress on your retinas, and also help protect them from sun damage.

Cantaloupe

This juicy, delicious orange fruit contains all of the vitamin A and C that you need in an entire day. Cantaloupes also have potassium, folate, magnesium, and vitamins B1, B6, and K crammed in there. This all translates into the following:

- **Energy production**—Since cantaloupe is a good source of B vitamins and potassium, it's awesome for supporting energy production, good metabolism, and stable blood sugar levels.
- **Eye health**—Because it contains both beta-carotene and vitamin A, cantaloupe is a perfect choice for eye health. The antioxidants also help protect your eyes from age-related conditions such as macular degeneration.
- **Immune function**—The list just goes on: The combination of vitamins A and C, along with the beta-carotene, protects you against disease-causing free radicals and supports good immune health, as well as reduces risk of cardiac disease, cancer, and stroke.
- **Lung health**—Studies are showing that a vitamin A–deficient diet can contribute to developing emphysema, especially in smokers or those exposed regularly to secondhand smoke. The amount of vitamin A in cantaloupe goes a long way toward protecting you.

Cranberries

Cranberries are red, so we know that that means—antioxidants! These little Thanksgiving treats should be appreciated and enjoyed year-round because, much like the other superfruits I've already covered, they're amazing for you. Some of the goodies in them include manganese and vitamins C, K, and E. Here's what else they offer:

- **Anti-aging benefits**—In addition to the antioxidants and other goodies that protect you from the damage free radicals can do, cranberries specifically contain resveratrol, a big hitter in the anti-wrinkle world.
- **Anti-inflammatory effects**—Cranberries are shown to provide important anti-inflammatory benefits to your digestive tract, starting at

the mouth and working their way down to the colon. This lowers your risk of all kinds of illnesses, including periodontal disease.

- **Heart health**—The antioxidants and anti-inflammatory properties of cranberries reduce oxidative stress and inflammation that can cause damage and plaque buildup in your blood vessels.
- **Immune support**—Exciting studies are indicating that cranberries may help change the severity of cold and flu symptoms. Is there perhaps a cure for the common cold right around the corner?
- **Urinary tract health**—Cranberries can help you avoid uric acid kidney stones, and their antibacterial effects can help prevent urinary tract infections.

Grapefruit

You've probably heard about the health benefits of grapefruit and its juice your entire life. Rich in vitamins C and A, grapefruit also contains potassium and B vitamins. Some of the specific benefits of grapefruit include:

- **Cancer prevention**—Grapefruits contain several different antioxidants that are beneficial in protecting you from cancers, including cancers of the lung, skin, breast, stomach, and colon. As a matter of fact, limonin, a particular phytonutrient found in grapefruit, actually keeps cancer cells from proliferating. These antioxidants also work to promote good health in general by preventing damage from free radicals.
- **Immune system support**—This one's a no-brainer. Because it's packed with vitamin C, grapefruit is excellent if you're looking for something to give your immune system a boost during cold and flu season.
- **Kidney stones prevention**—Because citric acid found in citrus fruits increases the pH in your urine, your risk of developing calcium stones is greatly reduced.

- **Lower cholesterol**—The pectin in grapefruit lowers both LDL levels in your blood and triglycerides.

Grapes

These little round orbs are a great fruit to throw into the juicer. Not to mention the fact that they're packed with antioxidants, they also have vitamins K, C, B1, and B6, manganese, and potassium. Grapes have a lot to offer:

- **Anti-aging benefits**—Because they're a rich source of the phytonutrient antioxidant resveratrol (among about thirty others), grapes are fantastic for wrinkle prevention and even reduction.
- **Anti-inflammatory benefits**—The antioxidants in grapes help prevent unwanted inflammation that leads to disease in a couple of different ways. They reduce the activity of pro-inflammatory messaging molecules and the production of pro-inflammatory enzymes.
- **Blood sugar regulation**—The phytonutrients in grapes are conducive to helping keep your blood sugar regulated.
- **Cancer prevention**—The antioxidants in grapes are particularly suited to helping reduce your risk of breast, prostate, and colon cancers.
- **Cardiovascular health**—This is probably the most studied area of grape benefits. Grapes in the form of red wine have been offered as the answer to the French paradox—a scientific question that addresses the fact that, though the French eat butter-laden, high-fat pastas, breads, sauces, and deserts, they are still among the most heart-healthy people on the planet. One of the explanations offered is the fact that they also consume red wine on a daily basis from the time they are young.
- **Cognitive health**—Consumption of grape juice has been shown to improve scores on verbal learning tests.

Kiwifruit

This sweet, juicy little green fruit packs more vitamin C than an orange and tastes like a pleasant mix of strawberry, banana, and honeydew. Kiwifruit's benefits include:

- **Asthma protection**—There's also an odd link between kiwifruit and a reduced incidence of respiratory-related problems such as asthma, wheezing, and shortness of breath in children.
- **DNA protection**—Scientists don't understand exactly how it works, but kiwis have an amazing ability to protect the DNA in the nucleus of your cells from oxidation.
- **Heart health**—People who ate two to three kiwis a day for four weeks reduced their potential for forming blood clots by nearly 20 percent compared to those who didn't eat kiwis. The fruit also reduces your triglycerides and protects your blood vessels and heart from oxidative damage.
- **Macular degeneration risk reduction**—The vitamin C and antioxidants in kiwifruit help protect you against age-related macular degeneration.

Lemons and Limes

I've already noted the fact that you can see the protection from oxidation that lemon juice provides just by squirting it on apple slices. Imagine, then, what this can do for your insides! Lemons and limes have similar compositions and nearly identical health benefits, so I'm grouping them together here:

- **Cancer prevention and treatment**—The antioxidants in lemons and limes work overtime to protect you from cancers of the skin, lung, stomach, colon, and mouth. In addition to helping prevent these cancers, limonin found in lemons and limes actually keeps cancer cells from dividing and proliferating.

- **General health**—The vitamin C found in these fruits is known to help prevent heart disease, many different kinds of cancer, and stroke.
- **Rheumatoid arthritis protection**—Studies indicate that vitamin C can help prevent age-related arthritis. Subjects in one long-term study who consumed the lowest amounts of vitamin C were more than three times more likely to develop arthritis than their C-consuming counterparts.

Oranges

Also packing a punch of vitamin C, oranges are rich in folate, vitamins B1 and A, potassium, and calcium. There are countless phytonutrients in an orange, too, including flavanones, anthocyanins, polyphenols, and hydroxycinnamic acids. In short, they're extremely good for you! Here's how:

- **Digestive health**—Studies are showing that oranges may help you avoid ulcers, and may also reduce your risk of getting stomach cancer.
- **Immune support**—Everybody knows that if you're getting a cold, coming down with the flu, or trying to recover from a hangover, you should drink orange juice. To delve a little deeper, vitamin C also prevents free radicals from triggering the inflammatory response that causes such illnesses as asthma, rheumatoid arthritis, cancer, and osteoarthritis.
- **Lower bad cholesterol and heart health improvement**—Vitamin C helps prevent the oxidization of cholesterol, which is what causes it to stick to the insides of your arteries. This helps prevent heart attacks and strokes.

- **Respiratory health**—Beta-cryptoxanthin, the orange-red carotenoid in oranges, is known to help keep your lungs healthy and prevent lung cancer.
- **Superior to a supplement**—The combination of nutrients, phytochemicals, antioxidants, and minerals in an orange all work together to provide many more health benefits than a vitamin C supplement alone can.

Papaya

This pear-shaped fruit with bright orange flesh and little black seeds has more health benefits than just about any other fruit listed so far. It has roughly three times the amount of vitamin C as an orange, and it's packed full of carotenes, flavonoids, B vitamins, pantothenic acid, folate, potassium, and magnesium. This benefits you in the following ways:

- **Cancer prevention**—The vitamin C, beta-carotene, and vitamin E in papaya are related to a reduced risk of colon cancer.
- **Heart health**—Because of the extremely high vitamin C content, as well as the vitamin E, folic acid, and vitamin A, papayas are extremely helpful in the prevention of hardened arteries and heart disease.
- **Inflammation reduction**—Vitamins A, C, and E, along with beta-carotene, are known anti-inflammatories and can help prevent asthma, arthritis, and similar diseases.
- **Immune system health**—Vitamins C and A both help boost your immune system so that you can fight off such illnesses as infections, colds, and the flu.
- **Vision health**—Vitamin A is great for your eyes, and papaya has lots of it!

Pears

Excellent for juicing, pears are tasty, but not so sweet that you can't use them with a few vegetables just to add a slightly woodsy flavor. They have vitamins C and K in addition to phytonutrients, and they help your body in several ways:

- **Eye health**—The vitamin C is helpful for preventing macular degeneration.
- **Hypoallergenic**—For some reason, people who are allergic to other fruits seem to be able to tolerate pears. This is one of the reasons that pears are popular as a baby food.

Pineapple

Packed full of vitamin C and manganese, pineapples also have significant amounts of vitamins B6 and B1, copper, and folate. Used to make many fruit juice cocktails, the sweet, citrusy flavor is known and loved throughout the world. When you're juicing pineapple, use the core and stem as well as the fruit because they're rich in bromelain, which I'll discuss here:

- **Bromelain**—This is a complex mixture of chemicals and is associated with benefits such as digestive comfort and anti-inflammation.
- **Energy production**—The manganese and B vitamins found in pineapples work to create an enzyme reaction that will give you an energy boost to help start your day.
- **Eye health**—The antioxidants found in pineapples contribute to healthy vision and can help prevent age-related macular degeneration.
- **Heart health**—Again, the vitamin C fights free radicals that would cause plaque buildup in your arteries.

- **Immune support**—The vitamin C works to keep you from getting ill. It also helps protect you from free-radical damage.

Plums

These juicy, delicious fruits are also good for adding to vegetable juice in order to sweeten it without adding a ton of sweet or obvious flavor. Rich in vitamins C, K, and A, plums also have tryptophan and potassium, as well as a ton of phytonutrients. Their advantages include:

- **Cancer prevention**—The antioxidants in plums help fight free radicals that cause cancer, aging, and other illnesses throughout the body.
- **Immune system strength**—I've already discussed the benefits of vitamin C for your immune system, and plums are chock-full of it!
- **Iron absorption**—There's documented research showing that plums make iron more available for absorption. This may have something to do with the vitamin C, but scientists really don't know.

Raspberries and Blackberries

Fragrant and sweet, with a texture that's perfect for everything from eating raw to making pies, raspberries and blackberries are incredibly nutritious both whole and juiced. They are actually members of the rose family, as well as being cousins to each other.

They're high in vitamins C, K, and E, manganese, magnesium, folate, copper, and potassium. In addition, raspberries also have omega-3 fatty acids—a group of necessary nutrients more commonly found in fish. They're also rich in tannins—phytonutrients that are responsible for much of the raspberry's antioxidant power. These two berries have some of the following benefits:

- **Anti-aging benefits**—Because of the antioxidants, manganese, and vitamin C, raspberries can help protect you from the damage caused by free radicals and oxidation. These include wrinkles, dull skin, and limp, dull hair.
- **Antimicrobial protection**—Raspberries can actually help your body fight certain fungi and bacteria that cause such issues as yeast infections, digestive issues, and some other illnesses.
- **Antioxidant and anti-carcinogenic protection**—Raspberries and blackberries are full of phytonutrients that fight free radicals known to cause heart disease, cancer, and many other illnesses and conditions.
- **Heart health**—The omega-3s in these berries are great for your heart as well as for your mood and cognitive function. What's interesting is that these fatty acids are rarely found in fruits and vegetables.

Strawberries

Delicious, nutritious strawberries. Rarely will you find a person who dislikes them, though you may find a few who are allergic. For the rest of us, though, these luscious berries make eating right so easy! They're packed full of vitamin C (one serving has 140 percent of your daily requirement!) as well as manganese, folate, iodine, potassium, magnesium, vitamin K, and—surprise!—omega-3 fatty acids. Some ways that strawberries help you include:

- **Anti-aging benefits**—Though this is also a relatively new area of study, strawberries are being associated with several different facets of anti-aging, including improved cognitive function, better balance, decreased risk of inflammatory arthritis and macular degeneration, and improved digestive health.
- **Blood sugar regulation**—This is a relatively new area of research. Regularly eating strawberries has officially been associated with a

decreased risk of type 2 diabetes. It's suspected that the polyphenols in strawberries play a key role in regulating your blood sugar.

- **Cancer prevention**—It goes without saying that the antioxidant punch that strawberries pack is extremely helpful in preventing several different types of cancer, including cancer of the cervix, colon, breast, and esophagus.
- **Cardiovascular health**—This is probably the best-documented benefit of strawberries. Because of the antioxidant and anti-inflammatory properties in the berry, there's a ton of protection from the oxidative damage caused by free radicals. They also help keep your arteries clean, your blood pressure normal, and your bad cholesterol low.

Watermelon

It may be listed last of the top fruits, but that's only because it starts with *w!* Watermelon is incredibly good for you, both in whole fruit and juiced form. It has an extremely high water content, so it's filling if you're looking for a nutritious snack. As a result, it's a great way to boost the water content of your juices without adding an overwhelmingly fruity flavor.

Watermelon is packed with vitamins C and A, potassium, and magnesium. It also has the phytonutrient lycopene, which is a carotenoid. Some contributions to your health may be:

- **Anti-aging benefits**—Arginine, an amino acid that's a product of the citrulline in watermelon, is being used to treat conditions, including erectile dysfunction, high blood pressure, insulin resistance, and type 2 diabetes. Arginine is also found in anti-aging creams, though there's not really much research that shows that it's topically effective.
- **Cancer prevention**—The lycopene in watermelon is linked with a reduced risk of cancers of the prostate, breast, colon, rectum,

and lung. There's also research that shows a decreased risk of endometrial cancer.

- **Eye health**—The antioxidants in watermelon work together to lower your risk of such age-related issues as reduced vision and macular degeneration.
- **Increased energy**—The B vitamins found in watermelon work with the magnesium and potassium to give you a nice energy boost that won't leave you feeling drained later.

In reviewing this list, many people may question why mango was not included. It was a tough decision because the wonderful-tasting fruit helps fight cancer, lowers cholesterol, helps clear up skin, helps maintain eye health, and alkalizes the body. However, it's difficult to work with and isn't readily available to everyone. It was for those two reasons that mango was left off the list, but if you like it and do have access, then by all means, use it!

Now that I've touched on the health benefits of the top twenty fruits, let's look at which veggies are best for you. After I cover that, I'll mention some herbs and spices, and then move on to some recipes. Keep reading—I'm almost to the best part!

(13)

TOP 20 VEGETABLES
AND WHY THEY MADE THE LIST

Though all vegetables are good for you, not all of them can be juiced. Nor do they all pack the same nutritional wallop. Some definitely stand out from others. The list below reflects the best of the best, so even if one of your favorites didn't make it, feel free to throw it into your juice blend anyway. Just because you don't see it here doesn't mean it's not good for you!

Asparagus

Considered a delicacy since ancient times, the tender stalks of the asparagus plant are packed with nutrients, and are best when used within a few days of being picked. Choose shoots that are between six to eight inches in order to get the best juice.

Nutrients include vitamins K, A, B complex, C, and E. Minerals found in asparagus include iron, copper, tryptophan, manganese, molybdenum, potassium, phosphorus, choline, zinc, magnesium, selenium, and calcium. It also contains protein! Health benefits include:

- **Antioxidant and anti-inflammatory benefits**—Asparagus has truly unique anti-inflammatory properties and is known to reduce your risk of developing Amyotrophic lateral sclerosis (ALS), type 2 diabetes, and heart disease.
- **Digestive health**—Because asparagus contains inulin, a carbohydrate that acts as a prebiotic in the large intestine, asparagus helps you absorb nutrients, and also reduces your risk of colon cancer.
- **Disease prevention**—The B vitamins in asparagus play a huge role in the metabolism of sugars, and thus, help regulate your blood sugar. They also control amino acids that may contribute to heart disease in high doses.

Beets

These colorful yet oft-scorned roots are rich in minerals and may be one of the primary reasons that many Russians live to be centenarians! Some of the nutrients include folate, manganese, potassium, vitamin C, tryptophan, magnesium, iron, phosphorus, and copper. They help in the following ways:

- **Cancer prevention**—The combination of antioxidant and anti-inflammatory properties in beets may make them beneficial in preventing cancers of the testes, prostate, lungs, stomach, nerves, and colon.
- **Detox support**—The betalain in beets helps in phase two of the metabolic process, which is where toxins are neutralized and excreted.
- **Eye and nerve health**—The unusual blend of antioxidants in beets is what really makes them stand out. In addition to the betalain, they also contain beta-carotene, manganese, vitamin C, and a rich blend of phytonutrients. They contribute to eye and nerve health.

- **Heart health**—Though studies are still in the early stages, beets are showing promise in heart disease prevention. The anti-inflammatory properties help prevent plaque buildup and other complications.
- **Optimal health promotion**—Beets, whether red or yellow, get their color from the pigment betalain, which is a powerful antioxidant and anti-inflammatory. It also plays a key role in cellular detoxification.

Bell Peppers

Bell peppers, regardless of color, are a great source of vitamins C, A, B complex, E, and K. They also have the minerals molybdenum, potassium, manganese, tryptophan, and magnesium. The wide array of phytonutrients gives them extra nutritive punch. Here are other ways they benefit you:

- **Eye health**—Because of their beta-carotene content, bell peppers are great for maintaining vision.
- **Health and wellness support**—There haven't been many studies specifically targeting peppers, but their high antioxidant and anti-inflammatory content suggest that they are beneficial for fighting many different types of cancer (specifically gastric and esophageal cancers), as well as other diseases related to chronic inflammation.

> **Did you know?** *Peppers are actually considered fruits because their seeds are on the inside. If you get really technical, many vegetables are actually fruits, according to the strictest definition of the word.*

Broccoli and Cauliflower

By the time you finish reading this, you're going to understand why your mother always told you to eat your broccoli! It's a superveggie if ever there was one, and cauliflower is right there with it. In addition to just about every major vitamin and mineral, they also have protein. Use these crunchy cruciferous veggies as much as possible! A few reasons why you should:

- **Cancer prevention**—The antioxidants and anti-inflammatory properties of broccoli and cauliflower help prevent many different types of cancer, including breast, prostate, colon, bladder, and ovarian. It also acts to protect your DNA.
- **Detoxification**—Broccoli and cauliflower have three special phytonutrients that create a unique combination. This pairing supports detox at every step of the process, which makes them perfect for a cleanse. They even help control the detox process at the genetic level! Though cauliflower only has about half the amount of phytonutrients that broccoli does, it is still a significant source.
- **Eye health**—The antioxidants, particularly lutein and beta-carotene, found in broccoli help protect your eyes from such diseases as age-related macular degeneration.
- **Vitamin D support**—The unusually strong combination of vitamin A and vitamin K (the pairing needed for vitamin D absorption) in broccoli makes it the ideal vegetable for people who suffer from a vitamin D deficiency.

Brussels Sprouts

Brussels sprouts have many of the same benefits as broccoli, which isn't surprising, considering that they are both cruciferous veggies. Brussels sprouts are actually a little better for you than their mildly greener cousins. Here's why:

- **Cancer prevention**—The numerous antioxidants and anti-inflammatory properties of Brussels sprouts make them excellent cancer fighters. Specifically, the vitamin K and glucosinolates work to keep your body free of disease, and the omega-3 fatty acids fight cancer as well.

- **Detoxification**—Brussels sprouts have four of the most crucial phytonutrients necessary for cell detoxification at all levels, including the genetic level. They're also rich in sulfur, which is a necessary component of the detox process.
- **Heart health**—Brussels sprouts are awesome at preventing inflammation that leads to plaque buildup and heart disease. They also have a component that may help prevent and maybe even reverse blood vessel damage. Finally, they help reduce bad (LDL) cholesterol, so they promote heart health from several different angles.
- **Other benefits**—Research is currently being conducted on how Brussels sprouts may help prevent other inflammation-related conditions such as diabetes, metabolic syndrome, irritable bowel syndrome, Crohn's disease, arthritis, and colitis.

Carrots

Bugs Bunny has been eating carrots for years and credits them for his excellent vision. There are many other health benefits to carrots as well. Plus, they taste good and add a nice smooth flavor to your juice.

Just one serving of carrots gives you 407 percent of your required vitamin A. You'll also be getting vitamins K, C, E, and all of the Bs, as well as potassium, manganese, molybdenum, and phosphorus. This adds up to some great advantages such as:

- **Cancer prevention**—Those same antioxidants and anti-inflammatory properties help protect you from a wide array of cancers.
- **Heart health**—Because they're rich in antioxidants, carrots help protect your cardiovascular system from free-radical damage and diseases caused by inflammation, such as plaque buildup.

Celery

This innocuous-looking, lean vegetable does much more than provide a decorative stir stick for your Bloody Mary. It's a great source of vitamin K, and also provides vitamins A, C, and B, as well as potassium, molybdenum, manganese, calcium, tryptophan, and magnesium. Health benefits include:

- **Heart health**—The phthalides in celery help keep your blood pressure low, and the vitamin C helps lower your cholesterol, which in turn keeps your arteries healthy.
- **Immune system support**—The vitamin C in celery helps prevent colds and the flu, and also provides protection from free radicals that cause inflammatory responses.
- **Urinary health**—The seeds in celery have been used for centuries as a diuretic. The potassium and calcium are important for helping your body regulate fluid balance and stimulate the production of urine.

Collard Greens, Turnip Greens, Kale, and Spinach

Turnip and collard greens, kale, and spinach all provide whopping amounts of vitamins K and A, and are also significant sources of just about every other vitamin and mineral. In short, they're amazing for you. Leafy green veggies are a bit harder to juice, but you really want to incorporate these into your cleanse for a variety of reasons. Because they do contain oxalates, use with care if you have kidney or gall bladder problems though. These greens help your body in the following ways:

- **Bone health**—The high amount of vitamin K helps keep your bones healthy. The calcium and magnesium are also great for skeletal health.

- **Cancer prevention**—The broad spectrum of antioxidants and anti-inflammatories makes these leafy greens awesome at preventing oxidation and other damage by free radicals. They also contain omega-3 fatty acids to fight free radicals.
- **Detox support**—Antioxidants and glucosinolates in leafy greens help with every step of detox including at the genetic level.
- **Heart health**—Just as with cancer prevention, the anti-inflammatory properties of greens keep your blood vessels healthy and lower your cholesterol. The folate in them helps prevent homocysteine buildup, which is a leading cause of heart disease.

Cucumbers

This refreshingly delightful, versatile veggie is nutritious as well as delicious, and is a must-have for anybody serious about juicing. It provides great flavor to both fruit and veggie concoctions, and the antioxidants in it gave it the final shove into the top twenty. Cucumbers are a good source of vitamin K as well as phytonutrients. Some of the ways they give your health a boost include:

- **Antioxidant powers**—Cucumbers are known for their extra free-radical scavenging benefits, as well as their anti-inflammatory properties. This helps with many different conditions, including arthritis, metabolic syndrome, and cardiovascular disease.
- **Cancer prevention**—Cucumbers are dense in phytonutrients known for their anti-cancer benefits. The cucurbitacins found in cukes block different signaling pathways required for cancer cell development. The lignans in cucumbers are associated with reduced risk of estrogen-related cancers, such as breast, uterine, ovarian, and prostate.

Fennel

This peppery, crunchy bulb is known for its excellent antioxidant properties. It adds a freshness to your juice that works well with many other veggies, including tomatoes, cucumber, and carrots. Its main nutrients include vitamin C, potassium, manganese, folate, molybdenum, phosphorus, calcium, magnesium, iron, copper, and vitamin B3. Here's what fennel has to offer:

- **Cancer prevention**—Phytonutrients, specifically anethole, is suspected to shut down the intercellular signaling system that stimulates tumor growth in the liver and possibly other organs.
- **Heart and colon health**—The folate and potassium in fennel helps reduce bad (LDL) cholesterol levels and keep homocysteine levels from elevating. This prevents plaque buildup and other oxidative damage. It also supports healthy blood pressure.
- **Immune support**—Vitamin C helps boost your immune system so that you can fight off colds, illnesses, and other diseases caused by germs. Vitamin C also fights free radicals to keep you healthy and free of disease.

Onions and Garlic

Pungently nutritious, onions and garlic pack quite the punch, both to the nose and to the system. You may need to play with your juice combinations a bit to work onions and garlic into the mix, but make the effort because they truly are good for you. They have vitamins C and B6, along with manganese, folate, potassium, and tryptophan. Their numerous benefits include:

- **Cancer prevention**—Entire volumes have been written about the anti-carcinogenic effects of both garlic and onions, and much of it has to do with the antioxidants and sulfides in them.

- **Digestive health**—Onions and garlic are both being studied for their effects on stomach ulcers and other digestive issues.
- **Immune health**—The antioxidants in onions and garlic work hard to keep you healthy by fighting off colds, the flu, and other illnesses that you may battle on a daily basis.
- **Iron metabolism**—Garlic specifically helps with the metabolism of iron by stimulating the production of ferroportin, a protein involved in the circulation of iron.
- **Mouth health**—Onions and garlic have antibacterial properties that may help kill the bacteria in your mouth that cause periodontal disease.

Red Cabbage

Though green cabbage is more commonly eaten than red, the red has all of the health benefits of green and then some. Because of the polyphenols that give it its color, as well as possessing a slightly sweeter flavor, shoot for the red. Here are a few reasons why:

- **Cancer prevention**—This area of disease prevention is by far the most researched and documented. There are even certain cancers that red cabbage is known to treat. This is due to the wonderful combination of antioxidants, anti-inflammatories, and glucosinolates.
- **Digestive support**—Cabbage juice has been used for decades to treat ulcers. Newer studies also show that the antioxidants and anti-inflammatories also help your intestinal lining and increase the good bacteria within your stomach.
- **Heart health**—Cabbage contains enzymes that help bind with bile that would otherwise bond with fat and cause high cholesterol.

Squash

For hundreds of years, squash has been used in simple rustic dishes and elegant recipes alike to add flavor, color, and nutrition. This yellow beauty has a texture similar to a cucumber, but it has a much higher nutritional value. Rich in vitamins A, C, and K, molybdenum, B vitamins, manganese, zinc, potassium, phosphorus, magnesium, copper, and tryptophan, squash also has protein and omega-3 fatty acids. Several ways it helps your body include:

- **Blood sugar stabilization**—Vitamin B complex, zinc, and magnesium are important for sugar metabolism, as are omega-3s.
- **Cancer prevention**—Because of the antioxidants and anti-inflammatory properties found in squash, oxidative stress caused by free radicals is minimized when you eat squash.
- **Cardio and digestive health**—The anti-inflammatory properties of squash are great for protecting you from such diseases as gastric ulcers, hardened arteries, and other inflammatory issues.
- **Eye health**—Vitamin A as well as lutein and zeaxanthin present in squash protect you from cataracts and age-related macular degeneration.
- **Prostate health**—Men who suffer from non-cancerous enlargement of the prostate gland (BPH) may receive relief from frequent urination by consuming the seeds of summer squash.

Sweet Potatoes

Looking for a way to get 438 percent of your daily vitamin A in one flavor-packed serving? If so, grab a sweet potato! Whether you opt for the orange or the purple variety, this tasty, dessert like vegetable has vitamins C and B complex, manganese, tryptophan, potassium, and copper. It also juices well, and adds flavor to any combination. Here are some reasons it's great for you:

- **Blood sugar stability**—It may seem odd that a starchy vegetable would help your blood sugar, but it does: sweet potatoes improve blood sugar regulation, even in people with type 2 diabetes. It's suspected that the protein hormone adiponectin plays a key role in this.
- **Eye health**—Because of the high vitamin A (beta-carotene) levels, these rusty tubers are just as good for your eyes as a carrot!
- **Heart health**—The anti-inflammatory properties and antioxidants found in the sweet potato help keep your blood vessels healthy and clear.
- **Nerve protection**—The phytonutrient fibrinogen, which plays a major role in blood clotting, can be harmful in large doses. It can damage nerve tissues and cause diseases such as multiple sclerosis. Sweet potatoes reduce inflammation and fibrinogen levels.

Tomatoes

Last but not least, is the versatile tomato. Bursting with flavor and nutrients, it's a great choice for a juice base, especially if you're new to the whole juicing thing. It's so easy to create delicious juices by starting with the tomato, because just about anything that you add to it is going to taste good. Even garlic and onion are more tolerable when mixed with tomatoes (think liquid spaghetti sauce!), so be sure to have plenty of these gems on hand before your start your fast.

Nutrients in tomatoes include vitamins C, A, E, K, and B complex, potassium, molybdenum, manganese, copper, magnesium, phosphorus, tryptophan, choline, iron, and protein. That translates to benefits for you in the following ways:

- **Bone health**—Lycopene, along with other phytonutrients, reduces oxidative stress in bones.

- **Cancer prevention**—Alpha-tomatine, an antioxidant, has been shown to alter metabolic activity in prostate cancer cells as well as lung cancer cells. Research is also being conducted regarding its effect on pancreatic and breast cancer cells, using lycopene as well as the a-tomatine, and results are promising.
- **Cardiovascular support**—This is where tomatoes really get a gold star: they are significant to heart health in two ways. First, they're packed with antioxidants that prevent plaque buildup and other damage caused by free radicals. Lycopene helps prevent the oxidation of fats in the membranes of your cells in your bloodstream. Second, lycopene and other phytonutrients in tomatoes regulate fats in the bloodstream, which keeps your cholesterol down. They also help regulate blood pressure.
- **Eye health**—Because of their beta-carotene and zeaxanthin content, tomatoes play a key role in helping to prevent such eye diseases as cataracts and age-related macular degeneration.

Now that you know what the best fruits and vegetables are and what they can do for you, let's cover some herbs and spices that will boost both the flavor and nutritional value of your juices.

14

SPICE IT UP—HERBS AND SPICES THAT MAKE JUICE SNAP!

Just like when you're cooking, you need to have your favorite herbs and spices on hand to bring your juices to life. In addition to adding flavor and dimension, these little miracle workers also boost the nutritional value of your juice. What follows is a list of the top ten herbs and spices so that you know what you're getting nutritionally when you add that zing.

Wheatgrass or Lemongrass

OK, so technically wheatgrass and lemongrass aren't herbs or spices. They're actually grasses, but a shot per day of either one is really helpful when juice cleansing because it can do any of the following for your body:

- Boost energy
- Fight free radicals
- Help eliminate toxins
- Help stabilize blood sugars
- Increase oxygen levels in the blood
- Promote healing

Note: Only certain machines will juice grasses, so if you're interested in using them, make sure that your juicer does before you buy it.

Basil

Like most leafy greens, basil has lots of vitamin K and minerals, as well as calcium and vitamin A. It also tastes amazing. If you want to add some freshness that is reminiscent of a good Italian sauce to your dish, throw a couple of basil leaves in. Work with a light hand though, because the flavor can get pretty strong.

> **Did you know?** Basil is being studied for its antibacterial properties. It has demonstrated the ability to inhibit strains of pathogenic bacteria that have become immune to antibiotics.

Cayenne Pepper

You can use cayenne fresh or dried, but you may have a hard time finding it fresh. The capsaicin that makes the pepper hot is known to reduce pain, promote heart health, and drain congested nasal passages. No surprise there, but it may shock you to learn that it's also known to prevent stomach ulcers, and many people use it as a weight-loss aid. You also get a dose of vitamin A from cayenne.

Cilantro

Also known as coriander, this has all of the phytonutrients that your leafy greens do. Cilantro helps lower bad (LDL) cholesterol and raises good (HDL) cholesterol. It also helps control blood sugar. Adding cilantro to your juice will lend it a spicy Spanish flavor (think salsa).

> **Did you know?** *Cilantro also has an antibacterial compound that's being tested for its apparent ability to kill salmonella.*

Cinnamon

Reminiscent of Christmas and Grandma's house, this lovely smelling spice is not only mentally heartwarming, it's actually clinically good for your heart. It's also beneficial for colon health and gives your brain and immune system a boost. It helps regulate your blood sugar levels, promotes healthy clotting, and has been shown to destroy bacteria and fungi such as the yeast Candida. Cinnamon is a good flavor pairing with vegetables as well as fruits, so go ahead and experiment with it.

Ginger

This zesty root has long been used to relieve gastrointestinal distress such as gas, motion sickness, and seasickness. It's also used to help with morning sickness for pregnant women and to boost the immune system in order to prevent colds. Its anti-inflammatory properties are also great for helping with arthritis pain and swelling, and it helps protect you from cancer.

> **Did you know?** *The gingerol found in ginger actually causes cell death in ovarian cancer cells. This is being studied currently to see how it can be used to effectively treat and prevent ovarian cancer.*

Horseradish

In addition to being pungently flavorful, horseradish spices up your health as well as your juice. There are so many benefits to this plant that the short of it is this: just use it. Rather than going into detail about each benefit, here's a summary of its greatest advantages. Adding horseradish to your juice protects against or gets rid of:

- Acne
- Arthritis and joint pain/swelling
- Bacterial illnesses
- Cancer
- Colds and flu
- Headaches
- Muscle aches and pains
- Respiratory problems
- Sinusitis
- Toxins (it's great for detoxing)
- Urinary tract infections

Oregano

Besides the aromatic flavor that oregano will give to your juice, it also brings cancer-fighting antioxidants and bacteria-fighting oils to your glass. As with basil, use a light hand until you get used to adding fresh herbs, because the flavor is quite prominent.

Peppermint

You've probably loved this flavor since you were a child. It's in chewing gum and candy, and at Christmastime, even candles and lotions smell like it. But did you know that there are some very real health benefits to eating (or drinking) peppermint? It's great for digestion and helps soothe a sick stomach. It's also rich in antioxidants and helps fight cancer.

Peppermint has microbial oils that kill bacteria, including E. coli, salmonella, and *Staphylococcus aureus*. Finally, the rosmarinic acid in peppermint helps with asthma and allergy symptoms. Since it tastes great, incorporate refreshingly cool peppermint to your juice whenever you can.

Watercress

This peppery plant is great for jazzing up your juice, and it brings several beneficial components as well. Here are just a few ways it helps your system:

- As a diuretic, it helps flush toxins
- Aids digestion
- Helps clear breathing passages
- Protects against cancer

For most people, watercress is perfectly safe, but if you're taking prescription medications such as chlorzoxazone, talk to your doctor first, because watercress changes the way that your body metabolizes the medication.

15

THE GOOD, THE BAD, AND THE UGLY

The entire point of juice fasting is to cleanse your system of accumulated toxins and garbage. This isn't an easy process for your body; you're probably going to experience at least some moderate side effects for the first few days of the fast. Though this is normal and actually a sign that you're on the right track, it can still be an uncomfortable experience. After a few days, the unpleasantness will fade and you'll begin to feel amazing, so stick with it!

The Bad (and Sometimes Ugly)

Headaches

Particularly if you didn't completely wean yourself off the caffeine and nicotine that you're used to consuming, you may experience headaches for a few days. As soon as your body adjusts to the lack of drugs, the headaches will subside.

Diarrhea or Constipation

The sudden lack of fiber in your diet may cause some temporary constipation. Some juicers recommend that adding a natural laxative to your juicing routine may be a good idea. On the other side of the coin, you may experience some diarrhea because you're not eating solid foods and all of the garbage is being flushed out of your digestive tract. If you have diarrhea for more than a day or two, or if it's severe, you may need to add just a bit of fiber back into your diet for a couple of days so that you don't become dehydrated.

Bad Breath, Body Odor, or Acne

These are possibly some of the worst side effects of juicing, at least from a social perspective. The other side effects are unpleasant, but at least you can deal with them mostly in private. Remember that the reason you're juicing is because you're trying to flush the toxins out of your body. The skin and the respiration process are two ways that your body gets rid of these toxins, so at least you know your cleanse is working. Relax, though, because these symptoms will go away within a few days as well.

Vomiting or Nausea

Again, you're flushing a ton of nutrients through your system with no fiber to slow down the process, so it may take a few days for your body to adjust. You may also be sick to your stomach because you're not used to the herbs or spices, or because you're undergoing some withdrawal symptoms. Finally, it may just be the sheer concentration of the juices. To minimize this risk, drink lots of water and dilute the juice by 50 percent.

Reduced Energy

For the first day or two of your cleanse, you may experience a drop in energy because you're not eating as many carbohydrates. Since the carbs that you *are* eating are being rapidly consumed and used, you may experience bursts of energy followed by a significant crash. You'll adapt after a few days, but this is the main reason that you shouldn't juice fast if you're diabetic. Also, it's one of the main reasons that seasoned juicers don't recommend consuming much fruit juice.

Side effects are normal for the first few days, but if they last longer than that, you should probably stop fasting and talk to your doctor. Just remember that you're experiencing the side effects because of the toxins and waste, not because of the juice. Stick with it! On the flip side, after the side effects go away, there are a few good changes that you're going to experience.

The Good

Increased Energy

Once all of the garbage is out of your system, you're going to feel amazing. Your energy levels will stabilize, and you'll notice that you have much more get-up-and-go than you did prior to the fast. This is the first sign that your cleanse is working. Your body is using all of the nutrients in the juice, and the solid foods and waste have been cleared from your system.

Glowing Skin

Skin care professionals will tell you that one of the main causes of acne is poor diet and inefficient waste disposal. Acne is your body literally pushing poisons out. Whether it's because your pores are clogged from the outside, or there are toxins forcing their way out from the inside, acne is essentially infection leaving your body. Once all of the toxins are out of your system, your skin will look great.

Mental Clarity

This is yet another side effect of a toxin-free body. Also, because you're not using a ton of energy for the digestive process, you have more energy left for other bodily functions, including the brain.

Weight Loss

It's only natural that you're going to be losing some weight, particularly if you're overweight when you start your fast. This is going to happen because you're clearing all solid foods and waste from your body, and because you're taking in fewer calories and fat for a period of time.

> **Did you know?** *You are typically carrying around five to seven pounds of fecal matter in your colon alone at any given time. Especially if you don't have regular bowel movements, this can cause buildup of toxins that can make you sick. You'll clean nearly all of this out in the first two days of your juice fast.*

Miscellaneous Good Stuff

Because you're consuming so many excellent enzymes, vitamins, minerals, antioxidants, and phytonutrients, don't be surprised if aches and pains that have been plaguing you disappear. It's not uncommon for digestive problems such as heartburn and gas to go away, too. After all, you now have a squeaky-clean system that can function efficiently and properly!

TIPS FOR A SUCCESSFUL JUICE FAST

Too often when you read about fasting experiences, you come across one of two stories: Some people admit to cheating "just a little bit" by eating occasionally. Others brag about how they lost countless pounds in a week because they drank only extremely low-calorie vegetables. Neither one of these instances describes a correct, healthy fasting experience.

If you're eating food, you're not juice fasting. If you're drinking so little that you're losing a significant amount of weight in a short amount of time, then you're not fasting healthily. Read on for some tips to help you have a happy, healthy, successful fasting experience.

Drink Enough

If you're going to fast properly, you need to drink enough so that your body is getting all of the nutrients and calories that it needs to survive. That means that you need to consume at least 1,200–1,500 calories. Otherwise, your body can't function properly and you also run the risk of damaging muscle structure. Because most juice is fairly low in calories, you can basically drink as much as you want and not drink "too much," but you should consume *at least* one gallon of juice per day.

Dilute Your Juice

Because of the purity of nutrients in the juice, you need to dilute it with water. If you like the flavor of the juice just as it is, then drink a glass of water along with your juice. You need to drink equal amounts so that your body can efficiently flush the wastes and toxins from your system.

Diluting the juice may help keep you from becoming nauseated while your body is adapting to your fast. In addition to water, it's also acceptable to drink herbal teas, as long as they don't have any caffeine, sodium, preservatives, or artificial sweeteners.

Use Mostly Vegetables

Fruit juice is full of nutrients that are amazing for you, but it is also packed full of natural sugars. This isn't so great for a couple of reasons. First, without fiber, the sugar is going to be absorbed immediately and converted into energy. Also, vegetables are much more nutrient-dense than fruits and will flood your body with nutrients without the sugar rush and accompanying crash.

Try to limit fruit juice to breakfast only. If you really want to use fruit in your other juices, try not to use more than one fruit component per recipe.

Clear the Juice Fast with Your Doctor

Juice fasts, though good for you, are a traumatic event for your body. It's tough enough if you're completely healthy, but if you have any health issues at all, you need to talk to your doctor before you start a juice fast. Especially if you're diabetic or suffer from any other metabolic or eating disorder, this type of cleanse may not be right for you.

Make Your Own Juice

Store-bought juices have most likely been pasteurized, which means that most of the beneficial enzymes that are going to make your fast successful have been destroyed. Also, additives and preservatives that are often used to extend the shelf life of the juice are exactly what you're trying to flush out of your system.

Use Organic Produce

One of the benefits of making your own juice is that you control the quality. Since you're fasting to flush all of the toxins and waste from your body, you want to avoid pesticides and chemicals. If you don't use organic produce, peeling your produce before you juice it is recommended.

> **Did you know?** *Because organic farmers strive for the strongest, most perfect strains of produce in order to fight off disease, these fruits and vegetables can be nutritionally superior to their pesticide-laden counterparts.*

Drink Your Juice Immediately

Many of the live enzymes in your juice begin to die as soon as you peel the produce, so in order to get the absolute maximum health benefit from your juice, drink it immediately. If you make juice in advance to take to work or school, make sure that you refrigerate it in an airtight container. Also, since you're drinking your juice raw without pasteurization to kill bacteria, the Mayo Clinic recommends washing both your produce and your juicer thoroughly to avoid food-borne illness.

Incorporate Green Vegetables

In addition to having amazing health benefits, green vegetables are alkalizing and help keep your pH levels where they need to be. This means that your body doesn't have to expend the energy to regulate them and has that much more energy to heal itself.

Fast from Three to Five Days

You'll hear of people who "cleanse" for a day, but that's a brief fast, not a true cleanse. It's a great way to get some concentrated nutrients, but it does no good if you're trying to rid your system of waste and toxins. It takes about two days to empty your body of solid waste, and your body can't really start cleansing and repairing until that happens.

Some people choose to fast for weeks or even months, but this isn't recommended by most health-care professionals or nutritionists. After seven days, your muscles begin to break down because you need protein in order to build and maintain lean muscle mass. Therefore, the ideal timeframe for a juice fast without detriment to your body would be three to five days.

I've now covered just about all of the points that you need to know in order to juice fast successfully. From this point on, I touch on specific needs that you might like to address with a juice fast, and also offer lots of recipes to help you achieve your cleansing and fasting goals.

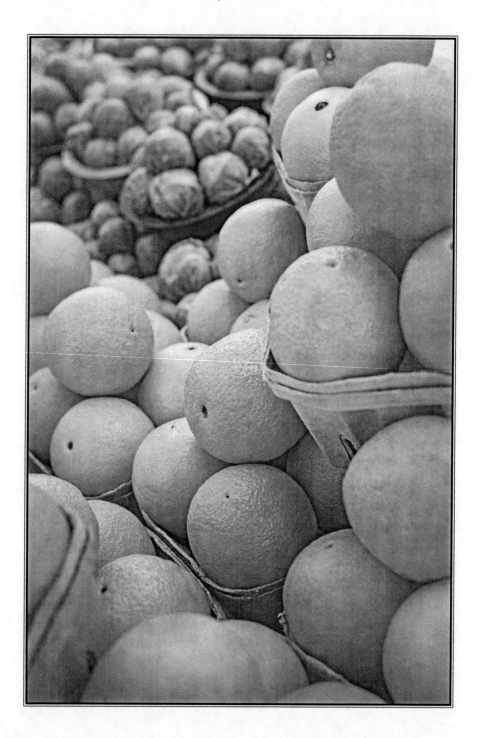

Getting Clean—Your Guide to Healthy Cleansing

GETTING CLEAN—YOUR GUIDE TO HEALTHY CLEANSING

As we learn to understand our bodies better, it's becoming increasingly obvious that toxins and chemicals are responsible for diseases that cause illness and death. We're all exposed to these toxins on a daily basis via food sources, our environment, and personal habits. As the toxins accumulate, the body can't function optimally. As a result, you might start to notice a lack of energy, decreased brain function, and just a general feeling of blah.

In order to get back your energy and your feeling of well being, you need to clean out the gunk. In other words, you need to detoxify your body in order to regain your health; juicing accomplishes this. If you just let the toxins continue to build up, you're inviting disease into your body.

Depending on what physical problems you face, there are different ways to cleanse. You may choose to participate in a general cleanse that treats your entire body, or you may want to target specific areas such as your colon, kidneys, or liver. Your personal habits dictate what kind of cleanse you need to undergo, so this is a purely personal decision—one solution isn't best for everyone.

In Chapter 17, I discuss the reasons for cleansing your liver and offer some tips and recipes to get you started.

In Chapter 18, colon cleansing is the topic du jour. I'll cover reasons that you may want or need to cleanse your colon, then go over some tips and recipes to get the gunk out. A good colon cleanse can also involve other parts of your digestive tract, so it may behoove you to do a total system cleanse, if you so choose.

In Chapter 19, I'll touch on the importance of a kidney cleanse, then review some methods and recipes that will help you along your way.

Cleansing is an independent and personal decision that you do strictly for your own health. Your doctor probably isn't going to prescribe it, and nobody is going to stand over you to make sure that you don't cheat. It's all about getting your health back, and your cleanse will be only as successful as you make it.

17

GET THAT LIVER CLEAN

Your liver performs literally hundreds of functions that are necessary for survival, and many of these involve filtering waste and toxins from your blood. Unfortunately, if you're not in the habit of eating healthy foods and drinking enough water on a daily basis, your liver is probably full of waste that hasn't been excreted properly.

The worst thing about your liver is that, if there's a problem, there are frequently no symptoms until the problem is out of control. Many liver diseases, such as cirrhosis, can't be cured or reversed, so it's crucial to be proactive when it comes to keeping this vital organ healthy. One of the best ways to do that is by keeping it clean so that toxins don't build up and cause disease.

There are some vitamins that really help keep your liver free of toxins, and you should try to incorporate those particular vitamins into your cleanse just to provide the extra boost.

For instance, thiamin, riboflavin, and niacin (vitamins B1, B2, and B3, respectively) assist in metabolizing such nutrients as carbohydrates and proteins. Vitamin B12 helps you keep from getting jaundice. All of the B vitamins help in one way or another so include produce such as potatoes, avocados, Brussels sprouts, broccoli, and cantaloupe in your juice fast.

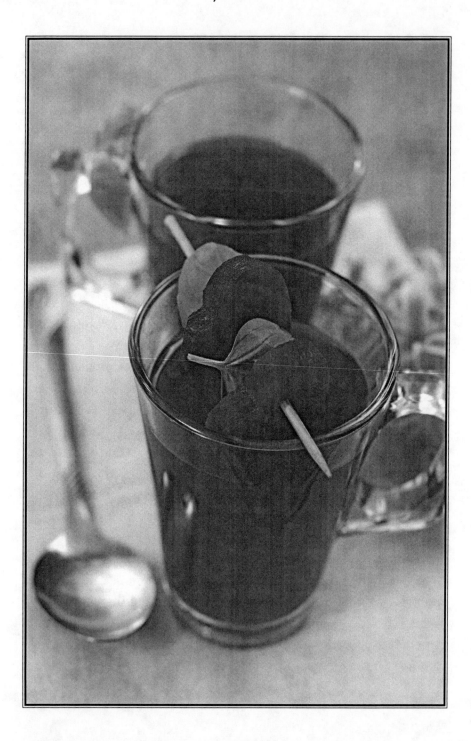

Vitamin C assists with iron absorption and helps flush fat and other junk out of your liver. Good sources of C include strawberries, broccoli, bell peppers, and citrus fruits.

Finally, acceptable amounts of vitamin E (one thousand milligrams or less per day) help your body process vitamins A and K, and can actually treat certain liver disorders. Vitamin E is an antioxidant as well, so it helps fight free radicals, too. You get vitamin E from avocados and leafy greens such as spinach and kale.

Now that you know what's good to incorporate into your juices for your liver's benefit, let's move on to some recipes.

Each recipe should yield about two cups of juice.

Green Beet Cleanse

Rich in vitamins A, K, C, and E, this drink is what your liver dreams about when it goes to bed at night. Oh, wait . . . your liver never gets a rest until you clean it out with this juice!

- 1 carrot
- 1 yellow beet
- 2 celery stalks
- 1 medium cucumber

Process all the ingredients in a juicer, and stir well to combine.

Veggie Vitae

When you're making this rich juice, it is helpful to process the cucumber last. Because of its high water content, it will help flush the juices from the leaves through the pulp and into your glass.

- ½ pound spinach
- 2 celery stalks with leaves
- 3 carrots with greens

- ½ apple
- 1 small cucumber

Process all the ingredients in a juicer, saving the cucumber for last. Stir well to combine.

The Dish on Dandelions

The Good: *Dandelions are extremely nutritious and you can eat the whole plant, from the roots to the flower. They provide nearly 40 percent of your daily vitamin C requirement, as well as 100 percent of your daily vitamin A and a whopping 500 percent of your vitamin K! They're also extremely low in sugar and have a small amount of protein.*

The Bad: *Dandelions aren't particularly easy to find unless you happen to have them growing in your yard. Be extremely careful picking them randomly, because most people think of them as weeds and spray them with pesticides. Always wash them before use, and don't pick them from unknown yards or along public sidewalks.*

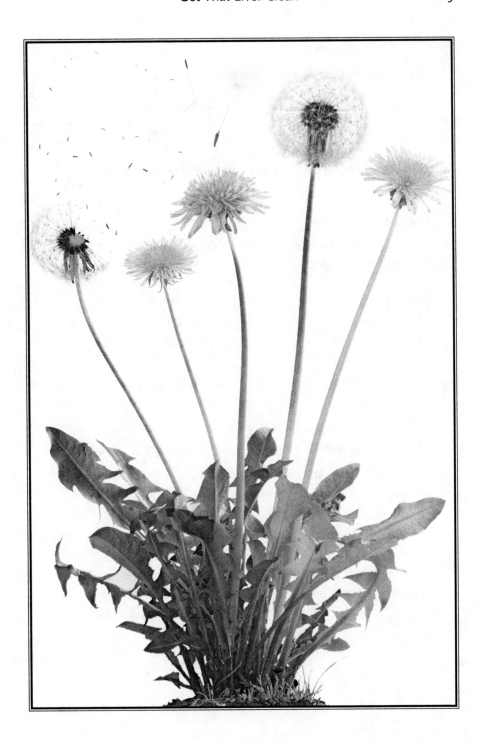

Beet Juice Supreme

The celery adds a nice lightness to this earthy juice.

• 2 beets	• 2 celery stalks
• 1 tomato	• 1 cucumber

Process all the ingredients in a juicer, and stir well to combine.

Dandelion Delight

Processing the cucumber's juicy flesh last helps push through more liquid and nutrients from the leafy greens in this bright-flavored juice.

• 2 celery stalks	• 3 kale leaves
• 2 cups spinach	• 1 cup parsley
• 1 cup dandelion greens	• 1 cucumber

Process all the ingredients in a juicer, saving the cucumber for last. Stir well to combine.

The Dish on Apples

The Good: *Apple juice has been used since ancient times for ailments related to a slow-functioning liver. The malic acid in the apples supposedly helps to break down solid substances such as heavy metals that accumulate in your liver.*

The Bad: *The traditional apple juice cleanse involved drinking large amounts of olive oil as well. However, that much fat makes your gall bladder contract and can cause a stone to get stuck, requiring immediate medical attention. This veggie juice is a nice, healthy alternative.*

Fennel and Greens

Typically found in many Italian dishes, fennel lends a nice peppery licorice flavor to this juice.

- 3 carrots
- ½ pound spinach
- ½ pound kale leaves
- 1 garlic clove
- ½ fennel bulb, including leaves and stem
- ½ lemon
- ½ teaspoon cayenne pepper

Process the carrots, spinach, kale, and garlic in a juicer, then the fennel, followed by the lemon. Add the cayenne to the juice, and stir well to combine.

Liven Up Your Liver Juice

Even the pretty color of this one will make your liver smile. This juice is packed with as much flavor as it is nutritional value, and will keep you coming back for more. By processing the apple last, you'll help push additional liquid and nutrients from the root vegetables through into your juice.

- 2 beets
- 2 carrots
- 1-inch piece ginger
- 1 apple
- ¼ teaspoon ground cinnamon

Process the beets, carrots, and ginger in a juicer, then the apple. Add the cinnamon to the juice, and stir well to combine.

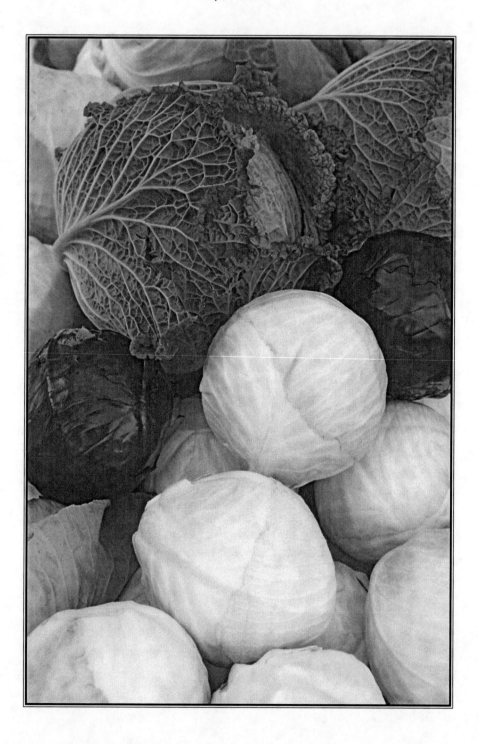

(18)

DIRTY COLON? CLEAN IT UP!

Are you suffering from brain fog, headaches, lack of energy, gas, bloating, or constipation? Maybe you're depressed or experiencing allergies for the first time. If so, it could be that your colon is so full of toxins, heavy metals, and waste that you're just not functioning well right now. Luckily, you can fix this, but you need to do it before your health is seriously affected.

Ideally, you eat good foods that are full of nutrients and fiber and your colon stays clean and healthy. Unfortunately, you probably don't eat perfectly all the time, and you're exposed to toxins on a daily basis from every angle. They're in the air, your food, and tap water. That processed, fatty food that's readily available everywhere you look doesn't help, either. What you need is a good juice cleanse to get your colon back on track. Let's talk about what you use to make your cleanse as colon-friendly as possible.

The first thing that you need is to make sure that you're getting plenty of is vitamin D. Your body gets this from exposure to sunlight, but it also needs vitamins K and A to absorb and process it. Vitamins C and E also contribute to colon health. Let's make some juices that make the most of these nutrients and are, therefore, perfect for your colon.

These recipes all yield about two cups of juice.

Cleansing Cocktail

Cabbage is traditionally used as a cleanser for your digestive tract. If you like spice, throw in a jalapeño pepper for a fiesta in a glass!

- 1 head broccoli
- 2 green bell peppers
- ½ head green cabbage
- 2 tomatoes

Process the broccoli in a juicer, then the bell peppers and cabbage, followed by the tomatoes. Stir well to combine.

Antioxidants Plus

This drink is reminiscent of a hearty vegetable stew. By processing the tomatoes last, you'll help push additional liquid and nutrients from the other ingredients through into your juice.

- 6 kale leaves
- 2 cups spinach
- ⅛ head cabbage
- 1 celery stalk
- 2 green bell peppers
- 3 carrots
- ¼ onion
- ½ beet
- ½ garlic clove
- 2 tomatoes

Process all the ingredients in a juicer, saving the tomatoes for last. Stir well to combine.

Orange Pineapple Chili

This sweet juice is perfect for breakfast. It's not only great for your colon, it's pretty good for getting rid of a cold, too.

- 2 carrots
- 1 orange
- ¼ pineapple
- ½ teaspoon cayenne pepper

Process the carrots in a juicer, then the orange and pineapple. Add the cayenne to the juice, and stir well to combine.

> ### *The Dish on Antioxidants*
>
> *The Good: Antioxidants bond with free radicals, effectively disabling them and carrying them out of the body through your waste. This prevents the free radicals from bonding with healthy cells and causing cancer, wrinkles, and other diseases.*
>
> *The Bad: Many people do their best to eat healthy foods that contain antioxidants but fail to drink enough water to effectively flush free radicals out of the system. Make sure you drink at least sixty-four ounces of water per day—even when you're juicing—so that your body can take out the trash.*

Sweet Spinach Carrot

You're going to be surprised by the sweet flavor of this juice, although the color may not be so pretty. It's stellar at cleaning your colon, though!

- 2 cups spinach
- ½ sweet potato
- 3 carrots

Process the spinach in a juicer, then the sweet potato and carrots. Stir well to combine.

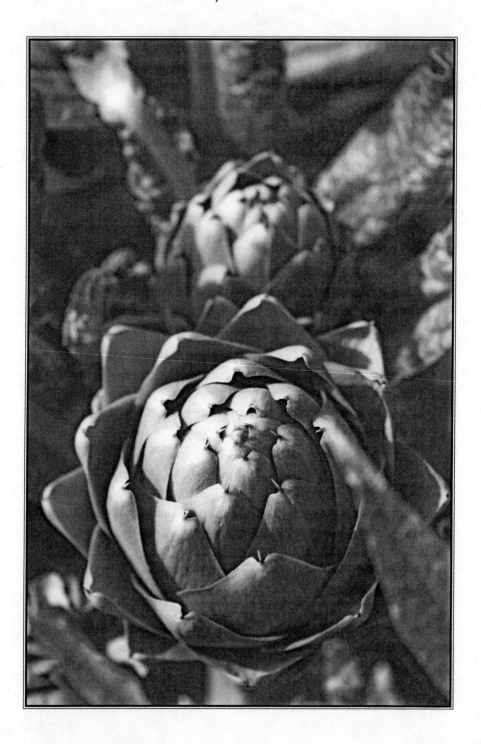

Broccolichoke Juice

Great for a vitamin boost and a bit of vegetable protein, this juice combination will not only satisfy your palate, it will do wonders for your colon. Processing the broccoli and artichoke with a little water here helps extract the most nutrients from them.

- 1 head broccoli, chopped
- 1 cup water
- 1 artichoke, chopped
- 1 carrot
- 1 garlic clove

Process the broccoli in a juicer, followed by ¼ cup water. Process the artichoke, then another ¼ cup water. Finally, process the carrot and garlic, followed by the remaining ½ cup water. Stir well to combine.

The Dish on Artichokes

The Good: *This odd-looking vegetable is absolutely packed with phenomenal nutrients. Artichokes are a good source of niacin and vitamins B6, K, and C, which makes them great for your colon. They also have more than four grams of protein apiece, and are low in carbs.*

The Bad: *Artichokes are a little hard to find in some parts of the country. In fact, that's why they didn't make the top twenty vegetables list. If you can find them, though, throw them into your juice whenever you can!*

Leafy Green Delight

The greens in this juice provide a veritable cocktail of vitamins and minerals. This is an ideal combination for detoxing and colon cleansing.

- 6 kale leaves
- 1 cup spinach
- 1 cup collard greens
- 1 bell pepper
- 1 garlic clove

Process all the ingredients in a juicer, and stir well to combine.

Cucumber Carrot Cocktail

This juice is an excellent one to take with you for lunch on the go, because the lemon juice helps prevent oxidation from occurring.

- 1 cucumber
- 4 carrots
- 1 apple
- 1 lemon

Process all the ingredients in a juicer. Immediately stir thoroughly but gently to evenly disperse the lemon juice without infusing oxidizing air.

Green Beast

This juice packs a nutritional punch that you won't find in many other combinations, and it also happens to taste really good. If you want to spice it up a bit, stir ½ teaspoon black or cayenne pepper into the juice.

- 3 kale leaves
- 1 cup spinach
- 6 Brussels sprouts
- 3 celery stalks
- 1 carrot
- 1 cucumber

Process the kale, spinach, and Brussels sprouts in a juicer, then the celery, carrot, and cucumber. Stir well to combine.

Pepper Sprout

This is a pleasantly refreshing juice with a bright, fresh flavor. It's great for lunch, because it gives you a nice nutritional boost without heaviness. By processing the celery and peppers after the basil, the herb's full flavor will come through in the juice.

- 1 cup alfalfa sprouts
- 6 Brussels sprouts
- 2 basil leaves
- 4 celery stalks
- 2 green bell peppers

Process the alfalfa sprouts, Brussels sprouts, and basil in a juicer, then the celery and bell peppers. Stir well to combine.

The Dish on Alfalfa Sprouts

The Good: Alfalfa sprouts are a good source of plant protein and vitamin K. They also have a pleasant, light flavor, and their mild juice offers a nice way to balance stronger flavors.

The Bad: There really is not any significant nutritional value in sprouts except for those touched on above. They can also be somewhat expensive.

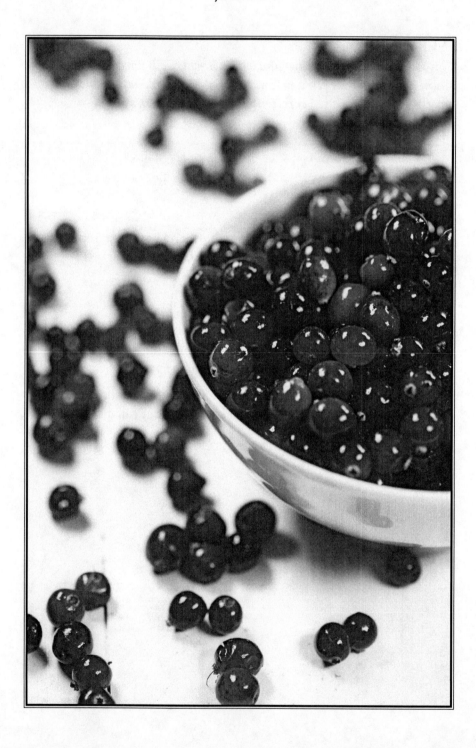

19

HELP YOUR KIDNEYS GO WITH THE FLOW

Your kidneys perform numerous functions that are necessary to your survival. As part of your urinary tract, they help filter liquid waste, but they also perform several other vital functions, including:

- Producing a form of vitamin D that promotes healthy bones
- Regulating the pH levels in your blood
- Regulating your blood pressure
- Regulating your water, salt, calcium, and phosphorus levels
- Stimulating red blood cell production

As you can see, these are crucial functions that you simply can't live without. As with the rest of your body, the best way to do that is by living a healthy lifestyle, including eating nutritious foods, limiting alcohol and other toxins, and exercising regularly. Poor living habits can lead to kidney stones, disease, and even failure, so take care of yourself!

In order to maintain good kidney health, you want to make sure that you're getting adequate amounts of nutrients that help reduce inflammation, regulate pH, and keep unnecessary strain from your urinary tract.

I've put together some recipes that are particularly good for your kidneys. Each one yields about two cups of juice.

Kidney Cleansing Juice

Dandelion greens are not only great for your liver, they're awesome for your kidneys, too! The lemon juice is also really good if you have calcium stones. This juice has a nice clean flavor due to the basil and lemon.

- 6 basil leaves
- 2 cups dandelion greens
- 3 celery stalks
- 1 lemon, peeled

Process the basil and dandelion greens in a juicer, then the celery and lemon. Stir well to combine.

> ### The Dish on Lemons
>
> **The Good:** *Lemon juice is great for breaking down calcium kidney stones. The acid in lemons disintegrates the stones and also creates an acidic environment that discourages new formations.*
>
> **The Bad:** *You don't want to let your blood get too acidic if you're prone to uric acid stones, so before using lemon juice as a kidney-cleansing agent, talk to your doctor.*

Cranberry Watermelon Cleanse

This recipe is great because the cranberries are antibacterial and, as such, are good for cleansing your kidneys and preventing infection.

- 2 mint sprigs
- 1 cup cranberries
- 2 cups watermelon

Process the mint in a juicer, then the cranberries and watermelon. Stir well to combine.

Watermelon Seed Tea

Though not technically a juice, this is one of the best cures known to science for helping avoid kidney stones, cleansing your kidneys and urinary tract, and stimulating underactive kidneys. If you're prone to kidney stones, you should drink this tea at least three times per week.

- 1 tablespoon crushed watermelon seeds
- 8 ounces boiling water

Pour the boiling water over the watermelon seeds and let them steep until the water cools to room temperature. Strain and consume.

Lemonade

This is actually used by top kidney stone treatment and research facilities to manage and prevent kidney stones. If you need to, add a bit of honey to sweeten it up a little.

- 4 lemons
- 1 cup water

Process the lemons in a juicer, then add the water. Stir well to combine.

Envy Juice

This juice is absolutely delicious. It has a nice spice, and the cucumber gives it a fresh, clean flavor that's sweetened by the apple and mint.

- 1-inch piece ginger
- 1 mint sprig
- 2 green apples
- 1 cucumber

Process the ginger and mint in a juicer, then the apples and cucumber. Stir well to combine.

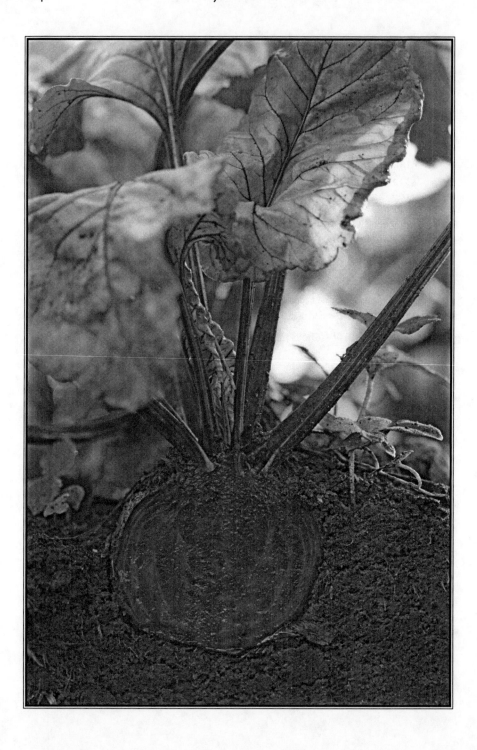

Cranbeet Watermelon

This cleansing juice will give you a nice energy boost without the crash, making it great at lunchtime or for an afternoon snack.

- 1 beet
- 1 cup cranberries
- 1 cup diced watermelon

Process the beet in a juicer, then the cranberries and watermelon. Stir well to combine.

The Dish on Beets

The Good: *The betalain in beets make them excellent cleansers because they help in phase two of the metabolic process, which is when toxins are neutralized and excreted.*

The Bad: *Beets are high in carbohydrates, so try to combine them with lower-carb vegetables, especially when first starting your fast. They're fine paired with fruits if you're just using them to add nutrients to a daily glass, though.*

Cranberry Lemonade

This juice is light and refreshing, especially when it's warm outside. The antioxidants and anti-inflammatory properties from the cranberries will make your digestive tract very happy.

- 1 cup cranberries
- 2 lemons
- 2 cups water

Process the cranberries and lemons in a juicer, then add the water. Stir well to combine.

Strawberry Banana Smoothie

You can't drink this during a juice fast because of the fiber in the banana, but if you're just looking for something really good for your kidneys, you can't go wrong with this smoothie! This one is processed in a blender for the added benefits the fibrous pulp offers.

- 6 strawberries
- 1 banana
- 1 pomegranate

Place the strawberries and banana into a blender. Seed the pomegranate, collecting its juice, then add the pulp and juice to the blender. Process for a smoothie, adding a little water as needed to thin the consistency.

Celery Pepper Sprout

Your immune system will benefit from this juice, as will your kidneys. The flavor is pleasant and light.

- 3 cups alfalfa sprouts
- 4 green bell peppers
- 4 celery stalks
- 1 cucumber

Process the alfalfa sprouts in a juicer, then the bell peppers, celery, and cucumber. Stir thoroughly but gently to combine without infusing oxidizing air.

Berry Melon Blast

The cucumber does a great job of cutting down on the sweet flavor and lightening up this tasty juice.

- 6 strawberries
- 1 cup diced honeydew
- 1 cup blueberries
- 1 cucumber

Process all the ingredients in a juicer, and stir well to combine.

The Dish on Blueberries

The Good: Blueberries are quite nearly the perfect food. Rich in antioxidants, vitamins, and minerals, you can't go wrong adding these beautiful blue fruits to your juices. For that matter, when you aren't juice fasting, eat a handful of them on your cereal or for a snack.

The Bad: The only downside is that because they're a fruit, they are high in sugar. However, there are studies being conducted indicating that something in blueberries may actually help reduce glucose levels in your blood.

Cherry Berry Lemonade

You can take this juice with you for lunch on the go without worrying about it losing nutrients, because the lemon juice slows the oxidation process. By processing the lemon last, you'll help push additional liquid and nutrients from the other ingredients through into your juice.

- 1 cup sour cherries
- 1 cup raspberries
- 1 cup blueberries
- 1 lemon

Process all the ingredients in a juicer, saving the lemon for last. Stir well to combine.

Plum Melon Chiller

This is a perfectly delicious juice for a hot summer day. If you're serving it to others, garnish with a mint sprig.

- 2 plums
- 1 cup diced watermelon
- 1 cucumber

Process all the ingredients in a juicer, and stir well to combine.

The Dish on Plums

The Good: *Plums are a good source of vitamins C, K, and A, which promote calcium absorption. Though there's not a big correlation between dietary calcium and kidney stones, there is a huge correlation between supplemental calcium and stones. Plums help you avoid stones and absorb your supplemental calcium.*

The Bad: *Plums do have a significant amount of sugar, and should therefore be used sparingly if you're trying to adhere to a strict cleanse.*

Guavaloupe Goodie

This orange glass of delicious nutrition is as easy to make as it is to drink.

- 6 carrots
- 1 guava
- 1 cup diced cantaloupe

Process the carrots in a juicer, then the guava and cantaloupe. Stir well to combine.

Green Shield

When preparing the asparagus for juicing, do so just as you would for cooking: hold each spear at either end and gently bend it until the stalk breaks naturally; discard the tough ends. If you want to spice this juice up, throw a jalapeño into the juicer or ½ teaspoon cayenne pepper into your glass.

- 1 bunch asparagus, ends trimmed
- 4 green bell peppers
- 6 celery stalks
- 1 lemon

Process the asparagus in a juicer, then the bell peppers, celery, and lemon. Stir well to combine.

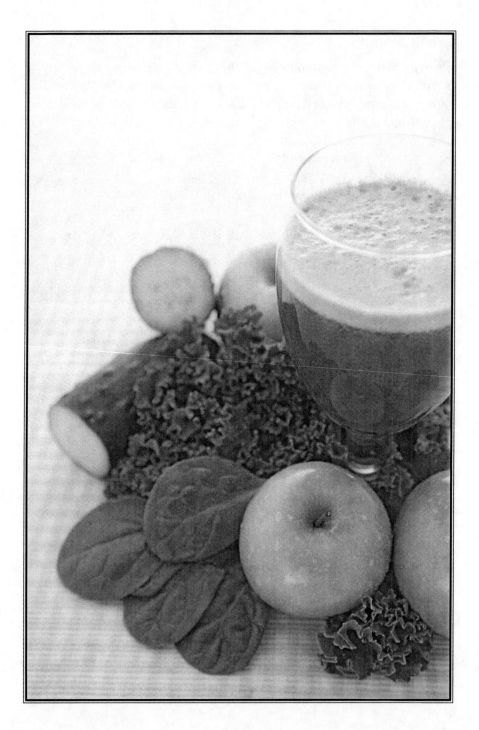

The Big Green Disease-Fighting Machine

THE BIG GREEN DISEASE-FIGHTING MACHINE

Though juicing is great for your entire body, there are some types of juices that are particularly good for specific organs or health needs. If you're juicing just to cleanse, then the recipes in the previous section are great. However, if you're looking to address a certain issue, you may want to target vitamins and nutrients that are known to treat that specifically.

Throughout the following chapters, I'll discuss a few common illnesses and concerns that you may wish to treat with beneficial juices. I've also composed recipes that are designed for the particular ailment you want to treat. Without further ado, let's get started.

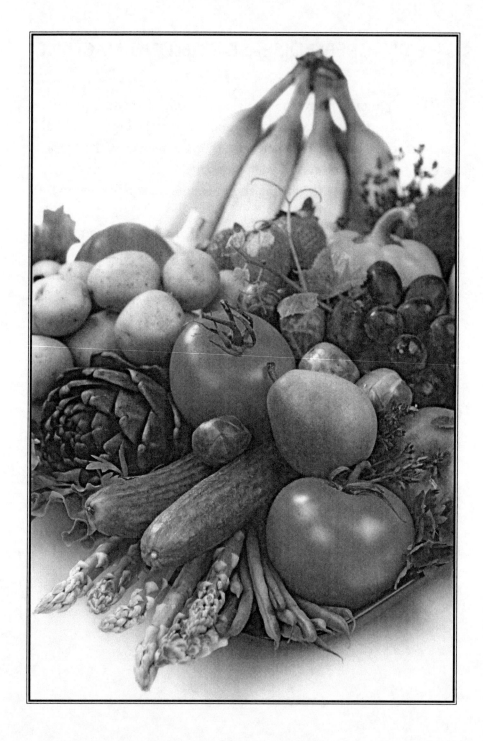

(20)

JUICING FOR THE HEALTH OF IT

You may be juice fasting for a particular reason, or maybe you just want a quick tonic to get rid of that wine headache from last night. Some activities, both good and bad, put extra strain on your body. Because of that extra strain, you may be experiencing headaches, muscle aches, nausea, or just a generally icky feeling. Regardless of your temporary problem, even if it's just a need for a great-tasting glass of juice, check out some of these tried-and-true recipes that are sure to cure what ails you.

All of these recipes yield about two cups of juice unless otherwise noted.

Hangover Juice

Magnesium, vitamin C, and calcium are necessary to get rid of that nasty day-after headache. You're probably dehydrated as well, so drink a big glass (or two!) of water with this. And if your hangover persists, drink another glass of juice.

- 1 cup cauliflower florets
- 1 cup broccoli florets
- 1 apple
- 1 orange

Process the cauliflower and broccoli in a juicer, then the apple and orange. Stir well to combine.

> ### *The Dish on Broccoli*
>
> ***The Good:*** *Broccoli is a good hangover cure because it's rich in magnesium, calcium, and vitamin C—all things that your body craves when it's trying to recover from a night of overindulging.*
>
> ***The Bad:*** *The juice may not taste wonderful, but remember that you did it to yourself, so take your medicine as easily as you took that shot!*

Snooze Juice

The number-one juice to drink if you really want to sleep is cherry because of its melatonin content. However, it's high in sugar and may cause energy bursts if you're juice fasting. This recipe contains melatonin and other nutrients known to reduce anxiety and induce sleep. As a bonus, it also tastes really great.

- ½-inch piece ginger
- 1 head broccoli
- 1 zucchini
- 1 carrot
- 1 apple
- 1 pear

Process the ginger, broccoli, and zucchini in a juicer, then the carrot, apple, and pear. Stir well to combine.

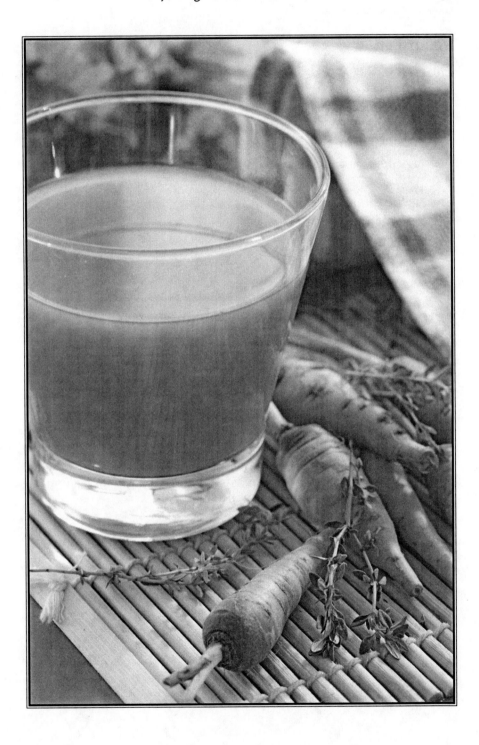

Reflux Redux

This is alkaline and will help soothe that heartburn. It's also soothing and a bit minty, so it won't be bad to sip. You may want to add a little water to achieve the right consistency; ginger is also a nice addition.

- 1 cup spinach
- 1 peppermint sprig
- 5 carrots

Process the spinach and peppermint in a juicer, then the carrots. Stir well to combine.

The Dish on Peppermint

The Good: *Peppermint has long been used as an aid for upset stomach. That's why restaurants and hotels serve mints after meals and before bed.*

The Bad: *Some people actually report a stomachache after consuming large amounts of mint, so as with all things, practice moderation!*

Peppermint Punch

Cool, fresh, and slightly sweet, this juice is a nice pick-me-up. It's really quite good if you add a splash of seltzer to it, too.

- 2 peppermint sprigs
- 2 apples
- 1 cucumber

Process the peppermint in a juicer, then the apples and cucumber. Stir well to combine.

Spring Tonic

Dandelions are known to treat everything from urinary problems to blood impurities. They are a diuretic as well as an anti-inflammatory, and are used to homeopathically treat such conditions as gout, constipation, and acne. When preparing the asparagus for juicing, do so just as you would for cooking: hold each spear at either end and gently bend it until the stalk breaks naturally; discard the tough ends. This recipe yields about four cups of juice, so you can drink it in two portions.

- 1 bunch asparagus, ends trimmed
- 5 whole dandelions
- 2 beets
- 1 head broccoli
- 4 carrots
- 2 apples

Process the asparagus in a juicer, then the dandelions, beets, broccoli, carrots, and apples. Stir well to combine.

Recovery Tonic

Rich in potassium, calcium, and antioxidants, this juice even has protein and omega-3s, so it's great to use as a recovery drink!

- 1 red potato
- 1 cup spinach
- 1 yellow squash
- 1 head broccoli
- 1 cucumber
- 1 celery stalk with leaves

Process the potato, spinach, squash, and broccoli in a juicer, then the cucumber and celery. Stir thoroughly but gently to avoid infusing oxidizing air.

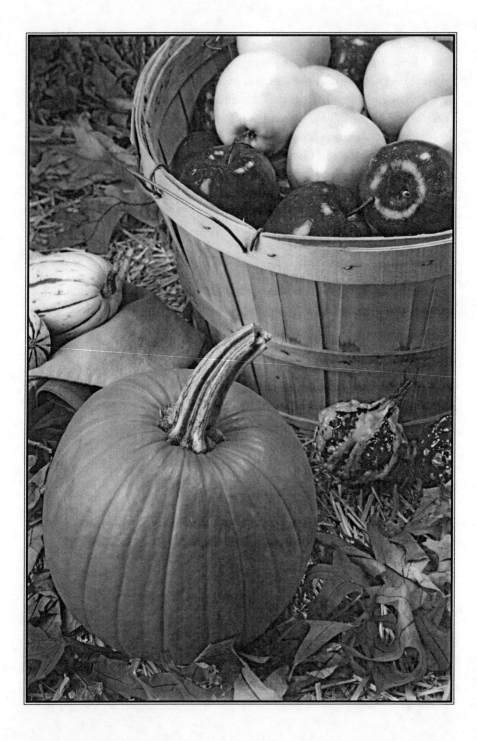

Harvest Helper

Rich in antioxidants as well as flavor, this juice will take you back to the soothing memories of grandma's house in wintertime. It's great for digestion, and good health in general.

- 2 sweet potatoes
- ¼-inch piece ginger
- 2 carrots
- 1 cup diced pumpkin
- 2 apples
- 1 teaspoon ground cinnamon

Process the sweet potatoes in a juicer, then the ginger, carrots, pumpkin, and apples. Add the cinnamon to the juice, and stir well to combine.

Belly Soother

The ginger and mint combination make for a happy stomach indeed. Since this recipe makes use of lime juice, you can take it to work with you if you're not feeling well, without fear of oxidation.

- 2 mint sprigs
- ¼-inch piece ginger
- ½ fennel bulb
- 1 apple
- 1 lime
- 1 cucumber

Process the mint in a juicer, then the ginger and fennel, followed by the apple, lime, and cucumber. Stir well to combine.

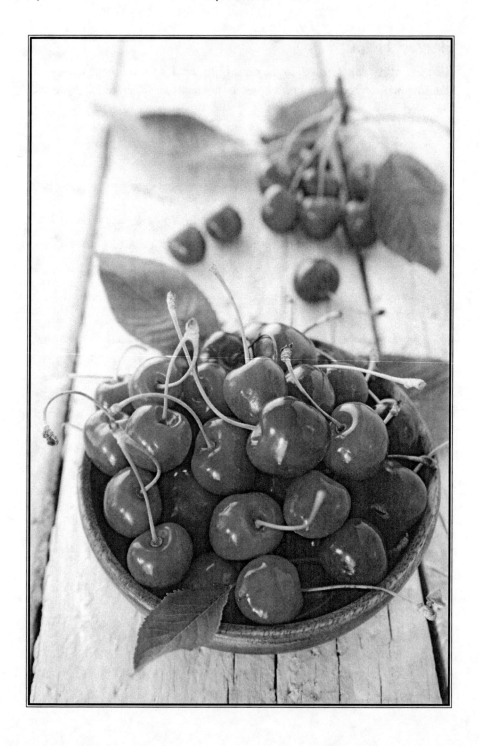

Slow Ginger Fizz

If you have an upset stomach, ginger is one of the best cures. It calms your stomach by relaxing the muscles around it.

- 3 kiwis
- 3 celery stalks
- ½-inch piece ginger
- 1 cucumber
- 1 apple
- 1 cup sour cherries

Process all the ingredients in a juicer, and stir well to combine.

The Dish on Cherries

The Good: *Cherries are packed full of more antioxidants than blueberries, and are also powerful anti-inflammatories. They're fat free, low in calories, and high in vitamins such as C and B complex. Eating twenty cherries may have the same pain-relieving and anti-inflammatory benefits as taking ibuprofen or aspirin.*

The Bad: *They are a fruit, so they have more carbohydrates than vegetables. However, that's really the only downside.*

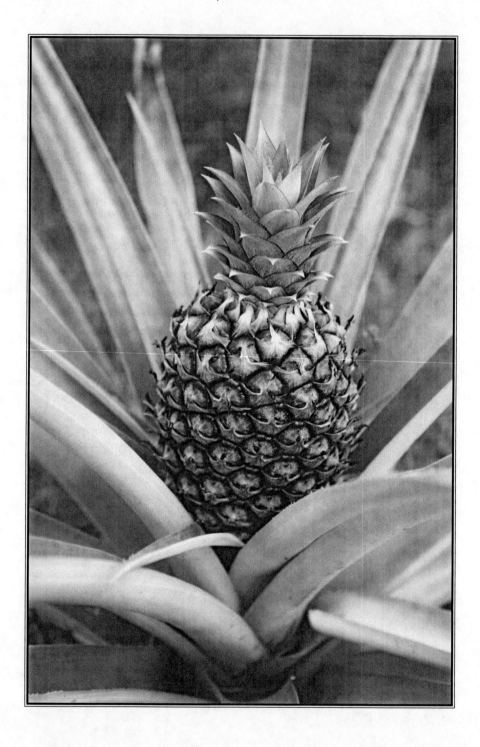

Allergy Helper

Since this one has lemon juice in it, it'll keep for a few hours without oxidizing, so if your allergies are bothering you, take some along on the go.

- ¼-inch piece ginger
- 2 carrots
- 1 pear
- 1 tangerine
- ¼ pineapple
- ½ lemon

Process the ginger and carrots in a juicer, then the pear, tangerine, pineapple, and lemon. Stir well to combine.

> ### The Dish on Pineapple
>
> **The Good:** *Not only is pineapple delicious, it also has some pretty amazing health benefits. It's obviously full of antioxidants, but it also has bromelain, an anti-inflammatory that works on sinuses and bronchial tubes. Pineapple helps reduce secretion from the mucous membranes, too. These all make it an ideal fruit to consume when battling allergies.*
>
> **The Bad:** *It's really high in sugar, which isn't so great if you're trying to either juice fast or hydrate to recover from a cold.*

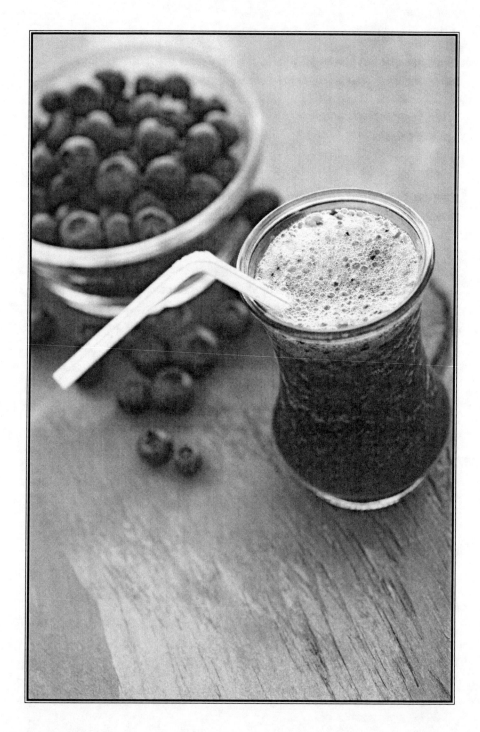

(21)

JUICING FOR ANTI-AGING—
JUICES THAT HELP KEEP YOU YOUNG

Billions of dollars are invested annually in the anti-aging industry. Researchers want to know what causes age-related illness so that they can find cures, cosmetics companies want to know what they can use as their next best wrinkle-fighting ingredient or "proprietary blend," and we average folks just want to know what we can do to look decent in the sunlight and survive past age sixty.

The best solution may not be found in a pill or a cream. Maybe it's as simple and inexpensive as walking through your garden or down the produce aisle of your local farmers' market. Our bodies are made to run as finely tuned machines, as long as they get the correct fuel. Unfortunately, more often than not, they don't. Instead, we stuff ourselves full of processed junk and artificial garbage, and expose our bodies to toxins, heavy metals, and other poisons.

In theory, good health and youthful looks are as simple as taking care of your body from the time that you're born until the day that you die. Of course, death is inevitable, but according to many philosophies, disease is not. Garbage in equals garbage out. In other words, you get from your body exactly what you put into it—no more and no less.

Incorporating quality juices with vitamins and minerals into your diet will help you get the excellent benefits they provide.

The biggest thing that you need in any anti-aging juice is antioxidants that will fight free radicals. Because daily living combined with a lifetime of exposure to toxins and other bad stuff has left you with cells that are freely oxidizing, you need the power of antioxidants to combat them. A good rule of thumb is that the brighter colored the produce, the higher they are in free-radical warfare artillery, not to mention flavor.

If you're looking for juices that can help you fight free radicals and meet the needs of an aging body, look no further. Just don't tell the cosmetic companies: it'll break their hearts (and their multibillion-dollar budgets).

The recipes in this chapter all yield about two cups of juice.

Green Apple Grape

This classic juice combo is fruity and pleasant. Note that some strict juicing fasts don't permit the use of honeydew because of the pulp that may leak through.

- 2 green apples
- 1 cup red grapes
- 1 cup diced honeydew

Process the apples and grapes in a juicer, then the honeydew. Stir well to combine.

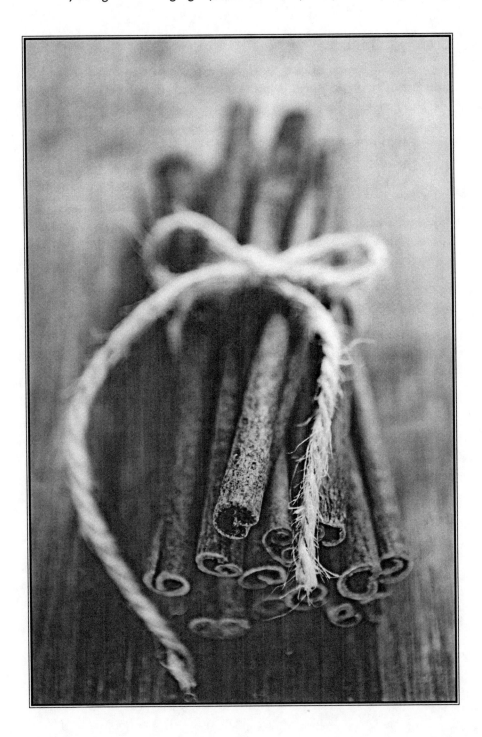

Granny's Go Juice

Because it's high in sugar, this juice is best saved to have as a treat or for breakfast. It's extremely high in antioxidants and has a ton of health benefits, though, so don't feel too guilty.

- 2 cups wheatgrass
- 3 carrots
- 1 beet
- 1 cup strawberries
- 1 cup blueberries
- 1 teaspoon ground cinnamon

Process the wheatgrass in a juicer, then the carrots and beet, followed by the strawberries and blueberries. Add the cinnamon to the juice, and stir well to combine.

> ### The Dish on Cinnamon
>
> **The Good:** *Cinnamon is an antibacterial that helps regulate blood sugar levels, promotes healthy blood clotting, and boosts your immune system and your brainpower.*
>
> **The Bad:** *Cinnamon can be a little expensive, and also adds a distinct flavor that doesn't mesh well with all juice ingredients.*

Super Popeye

This is a richly flavored juice that may not appeal to everyone, but it's absolutely incredible from a health and anti-aging point of view.

- 2 cups spinach
- 1 head broccoli
- 1 artichoke
- 4 carrots
- 1 cucumber

Process the spinach and broccoli in a juicer, then the artichoke, carrots, and cucumber. Stir well to combine.

Veggie Delite

This is similar to a Bloody Mary mixture with some kick to it. By processing the tomato last, you'll help push additional liquid and nutrients from the other ingredients through into your juice.

- 4 basil leaves
- 3 carrots
- 1 teaspoon grated horseradish
- 1 green bell pepper
- 1 tomato
- ¼ teaspoon cayenne pepper

Process the basil and carrots in a juicer, then the horseradish and bell pepper, followed by the tomato. Add the cayenne to the juice, and stir well to combine.

Ageless Beauty Juice

Keep yourself looking and feeling young by frequently whipping together this drink. The cucumber lightens the flavor of this juice a bit.

- 2 cups spinach
- ½ head broccoli
- ½ sweet potato
- 3 carrots
- 1 garlic clove
- 1 cucumber

Process the spinach, broccoli, and sweet potato in a juicer, then the carrots, garlic, and cucumber. Stir well to combine.

The Dish on Cucumbers

The Good: Cucumbers are packed with antioxidants and anti-inflammatories that help you fight arthritis, metabolic syndrome, and cardiovascular disease, as well as wrinkles. And its phytonutrients help you avoid many different kinds of cancer.

The Bad: There really is no downside to cucumbers. They're delicious, nutritious, and low in sugar. Make a point to eat them frequently!

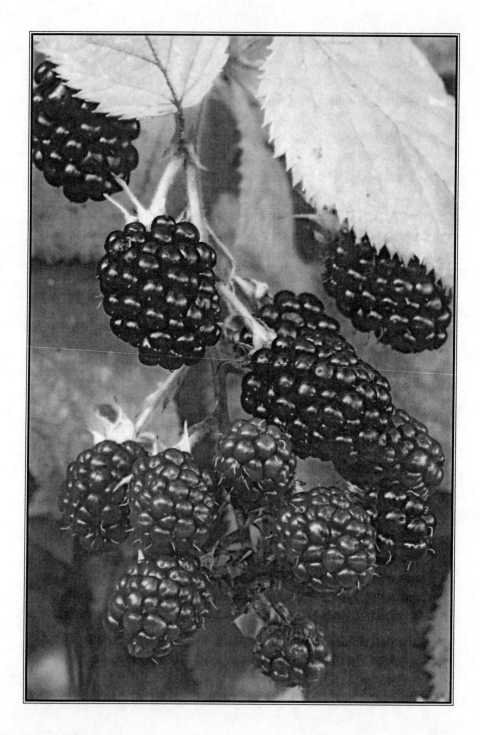

Fine Line Wine

This berry-packed recipe is an awesome choice for breakfast. Start your day with an antioxidant wallop!

- 2 apples
- ½ cup blueberries
- ½ cup blackberries
- ½ cup raspberries
- ½ cup strawberries
- ½ cup red grapes

Process all the ingredients in a juicer, and stir well to combine.

The Dish on Blackberries

The Good: *They're dark and they're berries. That should tell you already that they're packed full of antioxidants that fight cancer and disease. In addition to all their fabulous vitamins and minerals, they also have brain-boosting omega-3s.*

The Bad: *They're very high in sugar, and if you're eating the berry instead of juicing it, people with digestive issues may have a problem with the seeds.*

Antioxidant Punch

This is a cancer-preventing, wrinkle-fighting heavyweight.

- 2 celery stalks
- 1 cucumber
- 1 cup blueberries

Process the celery in a juicer, then the cucumber and blueberries. Stir well to combine.

Wrinkle Beeter

Once you get past the fact that the pleasant taste doesn't match the odd color, you're going to enjoy this juice!

- 1 sweet potato
- 2 beets
- 4 carrots
- 1 cucumber

Process the sweet potato and beets in a juicer, then the carrots and cucumber. Stir well to combine.

Collagen Juice

This one will boost your skin appearance. You may need to add a splash of water to cut the strength of the flavor a little. Also, you can add ½ teaspoon black pepper if you'd like to zing it up.

- 6 Brussels sprouts
- 1 beet
- ½ head cabbage
- 1 red bell pepper
- 1 head broccoli

Process the Brussels sprouts in a juicer, then the beet and cabbage, followed by the bell pepper and broccoli. Stir well to combine.

Snap Back Serum

This carrot-rich drink is great for your cardiovascular system as well as your vision. A dash of cinnamon is a nice addition here.

- 5 carrots
- 1-inch piece ginger
- 1 apple
- 1 lemon

Process the carrots and ginger in a juicer, then the apple and lemon. Stir well to combine.

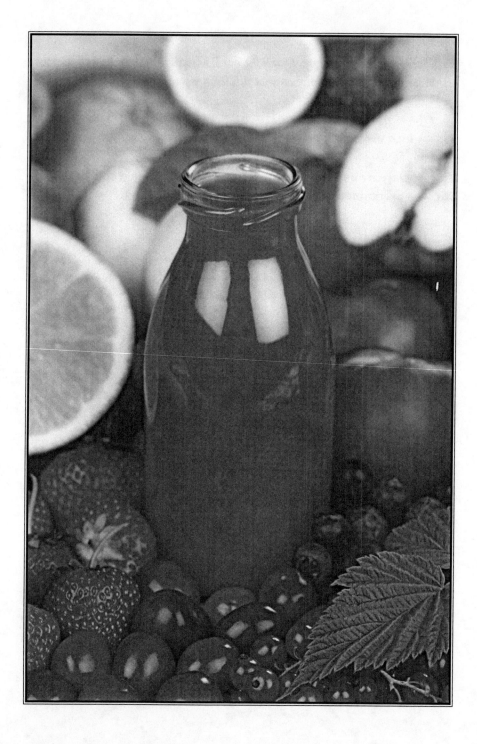

(22)

THE SMOKER'S GUIDE TO QUITTING—
HAVE SOME JUICE!

If you're a smoker who's trying to quit, nobody can tell you that it's
going to be easy. Smoking is a horrible addiction to conquer because
it has you hooked in more ways than one. On top of the nicotine depen-
dence, you also have to break the habit of having a cigarette in your
hand and mouth. This is particularly hard to do because it's not easy
to separate the behavior from all of the regular, day-to-day activities
with which it's associated.

Activities such as going to a restaurant, talking on the phone, and
driving aren't things that you are likely to give up, and since you probably smoke frequently while doing them, the two may seem inseparable.
When you combine the behavioral pattern with the physical addiction,
quitting smoking may seem impossible, but here's some great news:
it's not. It just takes some adjustment and conscious effort.

The juice recipes that follow can help you detox your system,
though they can't help with the smoking-associated habits. If you're
serious about quitting, though, try to alter your routine for a week or
more. Maybe take a vacation with nonsmoking friends or start an activity that's counter-indicative to smoking, such as swimming or going
to the gym. You're probably surrounded by people telling you to quit,

and they're right—but only you can know when you're actually ready to take that step toward a healthier you. The following juices will get you off on the right foot.

All recipes yield about two cups of juice.

Green Magic

This juice is packed with detox helpers working their magic in your body so you can start over fresh. By processing the celery and cucumber last, you'll help push additional liquid and nutrients from the other ingredients through into your juice.

- 2 cups spinach
- 6 basil leaves
- 6 Brussels sprouts
- 3 celery stalks
- 1 cucumber

Process the spinach in a juicer, then the basil and Brussels sprouts, followed by the celery and cucumber. Stir well to combine.

Strawberry Tomato

An orange-red hue means that this juice is flush with vitamins and nutrients that will protect your cells. There is some citric acid in the strawberries, so you may be OK storing this one for later.

- 3 carrots
- 6 strawberries
- 1 tomato
- 2 celery stalks

Process all the ingredients in a juicer, and stir well to combine.

Celery Apple Spritzer

A side effect of your smoking may be some issues with asthma: the apples in this juice will do wonders in helping reverse inflammation of and damage to your lungs.

- 2 apples
- 6 celery stalks
- 2 ounces seltzer

Process the apples and celery in a juicer, then add the seltzer. Stir well to combine.

Spicy Cabbage Stew

Great for fighting cancer, inflammation, and those extra pounds, this piquant juice will really wake you up. You may want to add ½ cup water to achieve the right consistency.

- ¼ head cabbage
- 2 green bell peppers
- ½ jalapeño pepper
- 3 green onions with stalks
- 2 celery stalks
- 2 carrots

Process the cabbage, bell peppers, and jalapeño in a juicer, then the green onions, celery, and carrots. Stir well to combine.

The Dish on Jalapeños

The Good: *The capsaicin in a jalapeño not only gives it its heat, it also has some pretty incredible disease-fighting abilities. It helps you combat cancer as well as common illnesses such as colds and the flu. It's a powerful anti-inflammatory, too, so it helps with arthritis. Finally, it's great for weight loss, because it can actually speed up your metabolism.*

The Bad: *They're hot! Depending upon your palate, you may not find the flavor of jalapeños pleasant.*

Pineapple Celery Pick-Me-Up

This juice is refreshing and great for a little boost of energy to get you through the afternoon. It tastes great, too!

- ¼ pineapple
- 3 celery stalks
- 1 cucumber

Process all the ingredients in a juicer, and stir well to combine.

(23)

CLEAR UP THAT COMPLEXION— HOW JUICING CURES ACNE

One of the things that most people don't think about is that your skin is not only an organ, it's also an exit for whatever your body may want to get rid of. Whether it's excess moisture, waste, or toxins, your skin is a big sieve through which your body excretes garbage. That's good since it's definitely better for the nasty stuff to get out, but the side effects can be really unpleasant and embarrassing (and obvious to others).

I've already mentioned the fact that your body simply wasn't made to run on processed foods, high amounts of simple carbohydrates, or an abundance of fat and protein. Sure, small amounts of all of those things may not be such a big deal, but you need to keep it moderate to avoid major issues. As a matter of fact, if you can eliminate the processed stuff altogether, you'll be much better off. There are no benefits to processed foods outside of convenience, and for the most part, all you're doing when you eat them is making your body work harder to clear the waste. One of the ways that it does that is via your skin, and the result can be acne.

When you're cleansing, your body flushes all of that waste out of your system, and that means though your skin. There are some juices

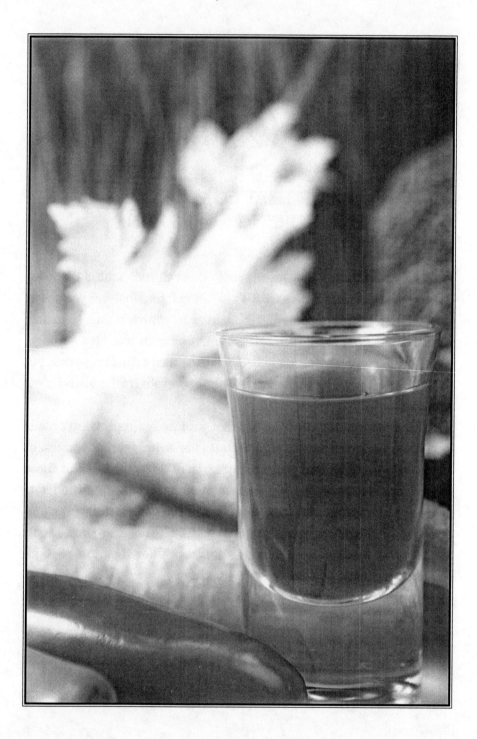

whose antibacterial and antioxidant properties really stand out from the crowd when it comes to fighting acne, and those are the ones that I've chosen to highlight in the recipes that follow. Mint, potatoes, and berries are particularly excellent, so incorporate them both juiced and whole into your diet as often as you can.

All recipes yield about two cups of juice.

Mint Magic

Kill bacteria and banish free radicals with this bright, herby juice. Since there's not much to it, this recipe is light and low in calories.

- ½ bunch parsley
- 4 mint sprigs
- 1 cup alfalfa sprouts
- 1 cucumber
- ½ lemon

Process the parsley, mint, and sprouts in a juicer, then the cucumber and lemon. Stir well to combine.

Red Refresher

This is delicious, refreshing, and fabulous for you, plus the color is beautiful. If you can't find pomegranate or just don't want to bother with it, cranberries make a stellar substitute.

- 1 beet
- 1 pomegranate (or substitute 1 cup cranberries)
- 1 cup diced watermelon

Process the beet in a juicer, then the pomegranate, followed by the watermelon. Stir well to combine.

Potato Purifier

This juice is simple to prepare yet very effective. Drink once per day for optimal acne treatment and skin care.

- 4 potatoes, red or white

Process the potatoes in a juicer.

> ### The Dish on Potatoes
>
> **The Good:** *The alkalizing power of potatoes helps balance your skin's pH, which is a leading cause of acne.*
>
> **The Bad:** *Potatoes are extremely high in starch and convert straight to glucose. If you're diabetic, you need to be careful with this juice.*

Green Restorative

Bring your skin back to life with this grassy-hued system cleanser. By processing the celery last, you'll help push additional liquid and nutrients from the other ingredients through into your juice.

- 2 cups spinach
- ¼ head cabbage
- 1 head broccoli
- 1 garlic clove
- 2 celery stalks

Process the spinach, cabbage, and broccoli in a juicer, then the garlic and celery. Stir well to combine.

Potato Melon Nectar

This juice is super refreshing as well as super for your skin.

- 1 sweet potato
- 1 white potato
- ¼ cantaloupe
- ½ cucumber

Process both potatoes in a juicer, then the cantaloupe and cucumber. Stir well to combine.

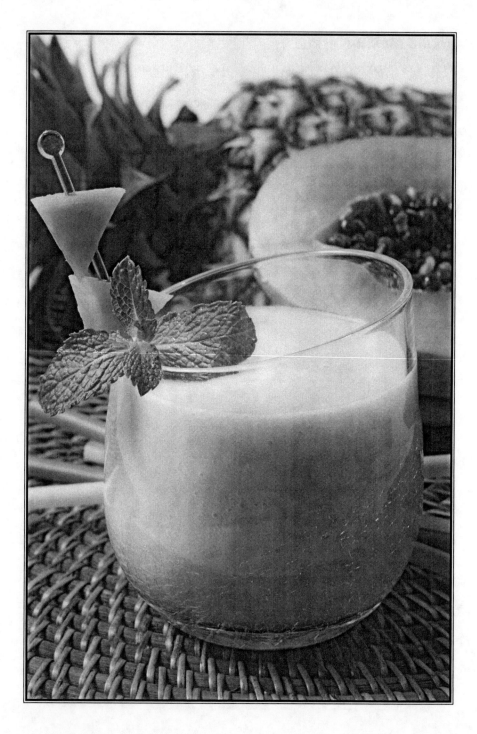

(24)

LEARNING TO FOCUS—CAN JUICING IMPROVE BRAIN FUNCTION?

The answer to this question, in a nutshell, is yes. Drinking fresh, organic juices, whether during a fast or throughout your average day, can definitely help you think better. The antioxidants in them help fight free radicals that destroy brain cells and prevent the flow of oxygen through the body. Juice fasting also clears all of the toxins from your liver and colon that may be causing imbalances, which contribute to poor concentration and brain fog.

On top of all of the repairs that juice can provide, it also rebuilds brain cells, nerve receptors, and other bodily functions that keep your noodle working. The nutrients in a glass of fresh juice comprise virtually every substance that your body needs to survive and thrive. If you don't believe this, try it for yourself. Give your body one week of freedom from all processed foods, excess fats, simple sugars, and other junk, and fuel it instead with fresh juice. I guarantee that you'll notice the difference! The following juices are particularly helpful for brain health.

All recipes yield about two cups of juice.

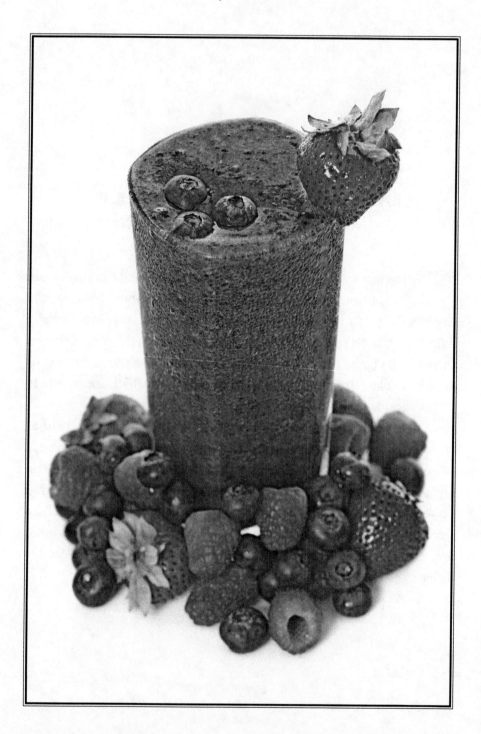

Mango Mint

Tropical and refreshing, you're going to love this juice, and your brain will get a major boost from it.

• 3 mint sprigs	• 1 mango
• 1 pomegranate	• 1 papaya

Process the mint in a juicer, then the pomegranate, mango, and papaya. Stir well to combine.

The Dish on Berry Combinations

The Good: *Any time that you mix berries into a juice or eat them for a snack, you're adding a handful of disease-fighting, age-defying deliciousness. Blackberries and blueberries are both packed with antioxidants that keep you healthy and improve circulation, brain function, and digestion.*

The Bad: *Berries are full of sugar, though at least it's natural fruit sugar. Still, if you're diabetic, this can be an issue.*

Berry Berry Cherry Juice

This antioxidant-rich fruit juice is best consumed early in the day. The lemon slows down oxidation, so you can take some of this on the go without worrying about oxidation.

• 1 cup blueberries	• 1 lemon
• 1 cup raspberries	• 1 cucumber
• 1 cup dark cherries	

Process the blueberries and raspberries in a juicer, then the cherries, lemon, and cucumber. Stir well to combine.

Grape Berry Guava

Guava and watermelon make this extra refreshing and especially so when it's hot outside. If you really enjoy fruity drinks, this is the juice for you.

- 1 cup raspberries
- 1 cup red grapes
- 1 guava
- 1 cup diced watermelon

Process the raspberries in a juicer, then the grapes and guava, followed by the watermelon. Stir well to combine.

Blueberry Blast

Make sure that you stir this juice pretty well to blend or else you're going to have cucumber juice floating on top and blackberry juice settled on the bottom.

- 1 cup blackberries
- 1 cup blueberries
- 1 cucumber

Process the blackberries in a juicer, then the blueberries and cucumber. Stir well to combine.

The Dish on Papaya

The Good: *Its antioxidants, including vitamin E, are excellent for memory as well as at fighting free radicals that cause other conditions and diseases. The potassium makes for good brain food, too.*

The Bad: *Papaya isn't available in all parts of the country, and it's extremely seasonal. It also gets most of its calories from sugars.*

Cherry Apple Chiller

Great for juicing or for serving to guests, this juice packs a nutritional punch that's hard to beat. Add the fact that it tastes wonderful, and you have a hit!

- 2 mint sprigs
- 2 apples
- 1 cup sour cherries
- 2 ounces seltzer water

Process the mint in a juicer, then the apples and cherries. Add the seltzer to the juice, and stir well to combine.

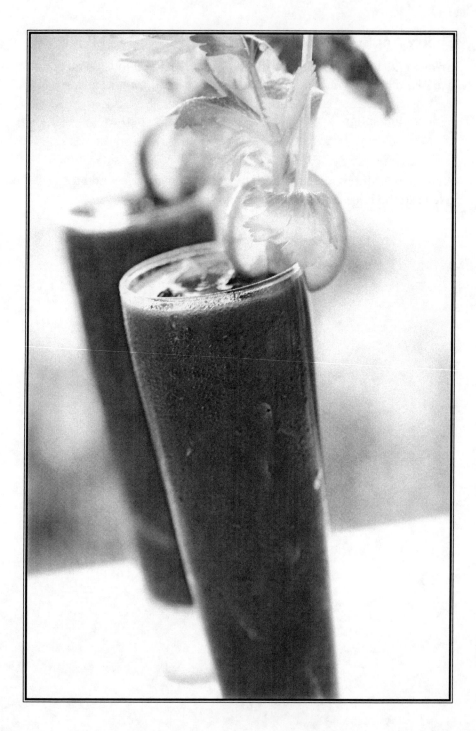

(25)

GET THE SKINNY—
JUICING FOR WEIGHT LOSS

One of the best ways to kick-start a weight loss program is with a quick juice fast. It'll flush the toxins from your body and make it that much easier for your system to process the healthy foods that you're going to be putting in it. A clean system also has more energy and is better able to utilize the oxygen that it gets during aerobic exercise. Finally, since you will be adding an exercise program to your weight-loss regimen (right?), your body needs to be functioning optimally in order to flush fats and build lean muscle.

Don't think of your new program as a diet, though, or even a weight-loss plan. Think of it as a new, long-term, healthy way to live. The weight loss that you'll experience from juicing and then eating healthy foods and exercising on a regular basis is just another side effect of a body that's functioning properly. Do it for your health as well as your looks. You'll feel much better and stick with it longer if you think of it that way instead of as a shortcut to a smaller pair of jeans. Here are some fitting recipes to start you off right. Good luck!

These recipes all yield about two cups of juice.

Skinny Italian

This juice is reminiscent of spaghetti sauce. It tastes great and is wonderful for you as well. You're going to love it! If you'd like, stir in ½ teaspoon black or cayenne pepper to really make it snazzy!

- 4 basil leaves
- 2 garlic cloves
- 3 oregano leaves
- 1 green bell pepper
- 2 green onions
- 2 tomatoes

Process the basil, garlic, and oregano in a juicer, then the bell pepper, followed by the green onions and tomatoes. Stir well to combine.

Skinny Margarita Juice

On those nights when the girls are all getting together, mix this up so that you don't feel completely left out. You'll find that it's a pretty good substitution.

- 4 celery stalks
- 2 apples
- 2 limes

Process the celery in a juicer, then the apples and limes. Stir well to combine.

The Dish on Limes

The Good: *The citric acid in limes is great for stimulating weight loss. It's a great antioxidant, too, so it helps you fight disease.*

The Bad: *Limes have a significant amount of carbohydrates from fruit sugars, so tread lightly.*

Citrus Serum

This juice is great for slimming down as well as beating a cold. Because of the high amount of citric acid, it's fine to take with you on the go without fear of oxidation.

- 1 orange
- 1 lemon
- 1 grapefruit

Process all the ingredients in a juicer, and stir well to combine.

Slender Sauce

The cayenne pepper and horseradish in this juice will kick your taste buds into high gear. Drink it after a trip to the gym to restore vitamins and minerals and keep the burn going.

- 2 celery stalks
- 3 tomatoes
- 1 teaspoon grated horseradish
- ½ lemon
- ½ lime
- ¼ teaspoon cayenne pepper

Process the celery, tomatoes, and horseradish in a juicer, then the lemon and lime. Add the cayenne to the juice, and stir well to combine.

Skinny Energy Shot

This combination of ingredients may not seem so appealing, but the metabolism boost you'll get from this juice will put any hesitation out of your mind. The lemon protects it from oxidation so that you can take it along with you.

- 1 handful wheatgrass
- ½-inch piece ginger
- ½ sweet potato
- ½ lemon
- ½ cup cranberries

Process the wheatgrass and ginger in a juicer, then the sweet potato, lemon, and cranberries. Stir well to combine.

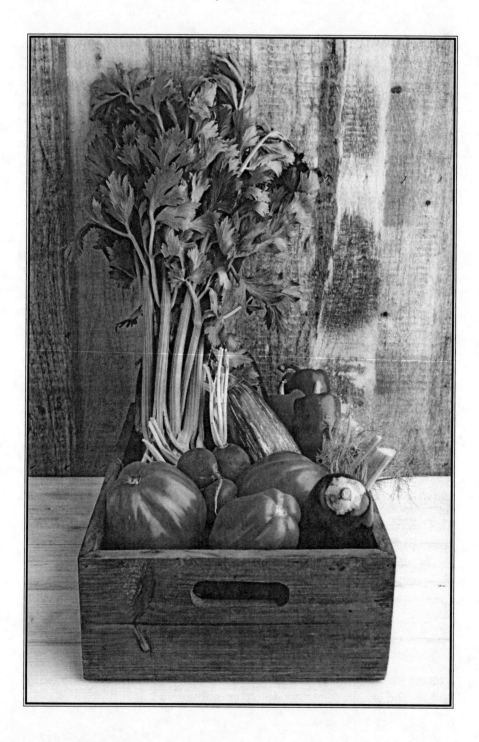

Slow Burn

This skinny juice is packed with nutrients, but without the calories. Feel free to add a whole jalapeño if you can tolerate the heat, because it's one of the main weight-loss ingredients.

- 3 celery stalks
- 2 tomatoes
- 1 lemon, peeled
- 2 carrots
- ½ jalapeño pepper

Process all the ingredients in a juicer, and stir well to combine.

The Dish on Celery

The Good: *In addition to all of the great antioxidants and nutrients in celery, it's great for any diet because it's a negative calorie food. Thus your body uses more calories digesting it than the celery actually contains, which means you actually lose weight consuming it!*

The Bad: *There really isn't a downside to celery. It's a great way to lighten up your juice and give it a pleasantly bright flavor.*

Spicy Lemonade

This is a cool lemonade with a kick! It's also another juice that you can pack up to go because the citric acid slows down oxidation.

- 3 lemons
- 1 cucumber
- 1 cup water
- ½ teaspoon cayenne pepper

Process the lemons and cucumber in a juicer. Add the water and cayenne to the juice, and stir well to combine.

Slimming Drink

This is a really nice drink that's bright and refreshing. If you want to, add some cayenne or jalapeño pepper for additional burn (in your mouth and around your waist!).

- ¼ cup chopped kale leaves
- ¼ cup spinach
- ¼ head romaine lettuce
- ½-inch piece ginger
- ¼ fennel bulb
- 1 celery stalk
- 1 apple
- ¼ cucumber
- ¼ lemon

Process the kale, spinach, lettuce, and ginger in a juicer, then the fennel, celery, apple, cucumber, and lemon. Stir well to combine.

Gingered Pear

A great all-purpose juice, this one's full of health-improving nutrients.

- ½-inch piece ginger
- 2 pears
- 1 apple
- 1 cucumber

Process the ginger in a juicer, then the pears, apple, and cucumber. Stir well to combine.

(26)

LOOSEN UP—JUICING FOR ARTHRITIS AND JOINT HEALTH

Arthritis, particularly rheumatoid arthritis, is a horribly debilitating disease that is frequently treated with medication that has side effects even worse than the arthritis. Many of the medications can cause liver or kidney failure, and oftentimes they don't even provide significant relief. If you're unfortunate enough to be a person who already suffers from other ailments, arthritis medications may not even be an option for you.

Fortunately, there are a few natural treatments that are actually exhibiting some signs of effectiveness with both pain relief and slowing the progression of the disease. Mainstream research institutions lay the cause of arthritis directly at the doorstep of the devilish free radicals, those rogue cells whose main goal is to steal the life from other cells. Fresh fruits and vegetables are rich in antioxidants—the nutrients that neutralize free radicals.

There are other fruits and veggies that have known anti-inflammatory and pain-relief effects and are thus great choices for inclusion in the juices that I've put together for you here. I sincerely hope that these help!

All recipes yield about two cups of juice.

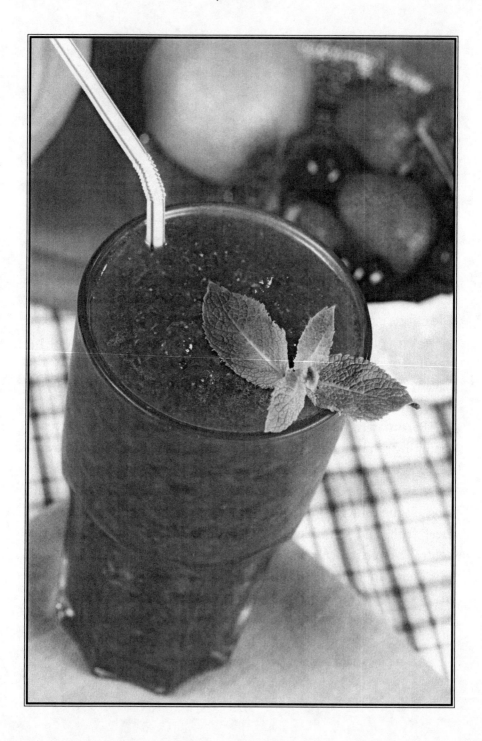

Pineapple Cherry Punch

Banish free radicals with this fruity punch. If you want to serve this while entertaining, add a spritz of seltzer.

- ¼ pineapple
- 2 plums
- 1 cup sour cherries

Process all the ingredients in a juicer, and stir well to combine.

Cherry Berry Mint Julep

The mint adds a nice touch to this sweet juice.

- 4 mint sprigs
- 1 cup cherries
- 1 cup raspberries
- 1 cucumber
- 1 apple

Process the mint in a juicer, then the cherries and raspberries, followed by the cucumber and apple. Stir well to combine.

Apple Mint Juice

This juice comes out an odd color, but it's extremely flavorful and very good for you.

- 4 mint sprigs
- 2 apples
- 1 carrot
- 1 pear
- 2 kiwis

Process the mint in a juicer, then the apples, carrot, and pear, followed by the kiwis. Stir well to combine.

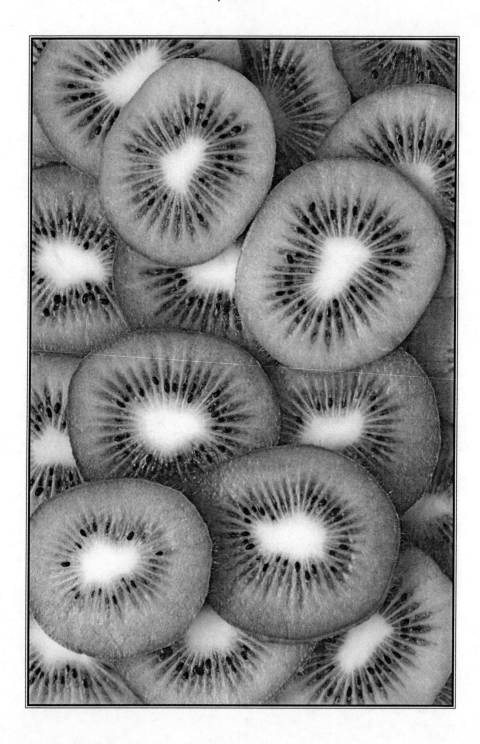

Potato Pineapple Splash

Ginger is an excellent anti-inflammatory, and the kiwi protects your heart and DNA. Add them together and you have a recipe for a healthy, long life.

- 1 red potato
- ¼-inch piece ginger
- 2 kiwis
- ¼ pineapple

Process the potato and ginger in a juicer, then the kiwis and pineapple. Stir well to combine.

The Dish on Kiwis

The Good: *Scientists don't totally understand it, but kiwis have an odd way of protecting the DNA in your cells from damage. They also have antioxidant and anti-inflammatory properties that are really good for managing arthritis.*

The Bad: *Kiwis have a significant amount of sugar, and are hard to find during certain seasons and in some locations. They also can be expensive.*

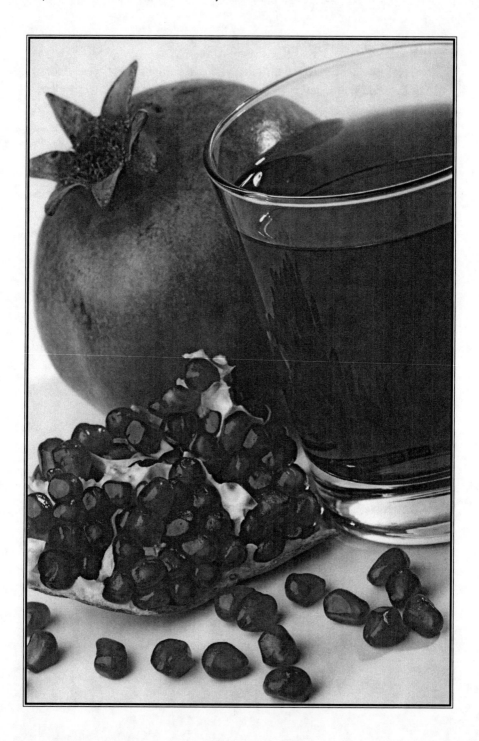

Pomegranate Cherry Juice

Drink your arthritis away with this juice rich with anti-inflammatories. If you can't find pomegranate, cranberries make a great substitute.

- 2 beets
- ½ cup blackberries
- 1 pomegranate (or substitute 1 cup cranberries)

- ½ cup sour cherries
- 2 kiwis

Process the beets and blackberries in a juicer, then the pomegranate, cherries, and kiwis. Stir well to combine.

The Dish on Pomegranates

The Good: *Pomegranates are a relatively new addition to the Western fruit scene. The health benefits of this seedy red fruit are proving to be numerous. They're full of antioxidants and anti-inflammatories that make them a stellar choice for arthritis treatment.*

The Bad: *Pomegranates have high sugar content and are difficult to find in many locations.*

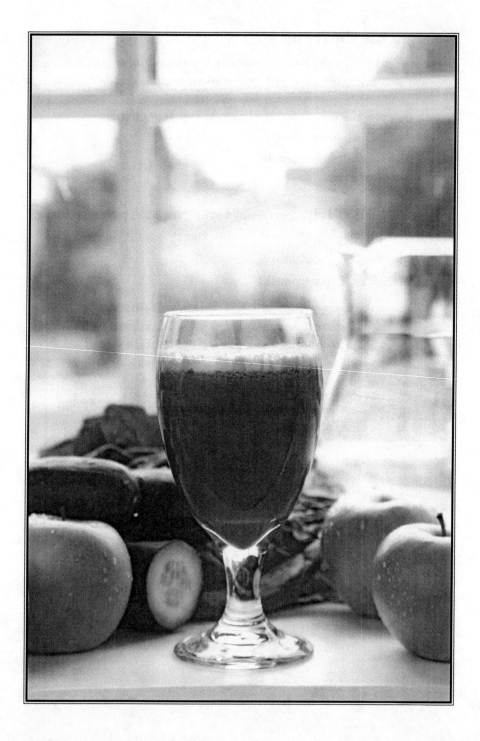

(27)

THE CURE FOR THE COMMON COLD?

Yep, you heard right. I'm suggesting that natural fruits and vegetables hold the key to the mysterious cure that's eluded the greatest minds on the planet for centuries. The answer's been sitting right there on the plate in front of you, or in the basket on Grandma's dining room table. The antioxidants found in all of those juicy, beautifully colorful, shiny fruits and veggies may actually be able to cure the common cold.

Turns out we've been looking in the wrong place for the solution: instead of the petri dish, we should have been looking in the garden! The antioxidants, anti-inflammatories, and pro-health goodies found in organic produce do an excellent job of helping boost your immune system so that you don't get a cold to begin with. If you do get one, vitamin C will help you kick it to the curb quickly. I've compiled juices that are packed with vitamins and minerals to help you avoid that nuisance of a cold altogether.

All recipes yield about two cups of juice.

Green Meanie

This is tasty and will chase your cold away in no time.

- 1 cup spinach
- 4 kale leaves
- 6 Brussels sprouts
- 2 green onions with stalks
- 1 jalapeño pepper
- 2 garlic cloves
- 1 lime
- 1 cucumber

Process the spinach, kale, Brussels sprouts, and green onions in a juicer, then the jalapeño, garlic, and lime, followed by the cucumber. Stir well to combine.

Simply Orange

An incredibly simple recipe, but some things are perfect just the way they are!

- 3 whole oranges

Process the oranges in a juicer.

Citrus Sparkler

If you're battling a nasty illness, this drink is sure to boost your system and your mood!

- ¼ pineapple
- 1 orange
- 1 lemon
- 2 ounces seltzer water

Process the pineapple, orange, and lemon in a juicer, then add the seltzer to the juice. Stir well to combine.

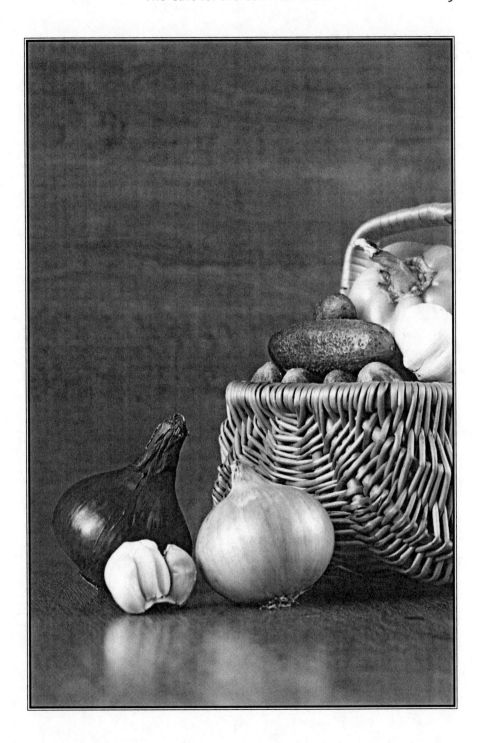

Unkissable but Cured

As the name suggests, you may not win many friends with your breath after drinking this (and thus it may not be the best choice for bringing to work), but your body will definitely appreciate it.

- 1 cup spinach
- 1 onion
- 1 jalapeño pepper
- 4 carrots
- 2 green bell peppers
- 2 garlic cloves
- 1 cucumber

Process the spinach, onion, and jalapeño in a juicer, then the carrots, bell peppers, and garlic, followed by the cucumber. Stir well to combine.

The Dish on Garlic

The Good: *From a nutritional standpoint, garlic is one of the most perfect foods that you can incorporate into your diet. It's full of antioxidants and anti-inflammatories. It boosts your immune system, prevents cancer, and helps with digestion. It's also an antibacterial.*

The Bad: *The only real downside to garlic is the aroma and effect it has on your breath. It can also be a little sticky to work with.*

Gesundheit Gazpacho

Drink the sneezes away with this restorative juice.

- 2 tomatoes
- 1 green bell pepper
- 2 green onions
- 1 garlic clove

Process all the ingredients in a juicer, and stir well to combine.

Muscle Ache Drink

The ingredient combination here is perfect for a post-workout recharge, or just an immunity boost when you're feeling blah.

- 1 cup spinach
- 6 kale leaves
- 1 head broccoli
- 4 carrots
- 1 apple

Process the spinach and kale in a juicer, then the broccoli and carrots, followed by the apple. Stir well to combine.

Ginger Tea

Great for settling the stomach when you have the flu, this tea also ensures you stay well hydrated.

- 4 cups water
- 2-inch piece ginger
- ¼ lemon

Bring the water to a boil and add the ginger. Boil for fifteen to twenty minutes. Strain the tea, discarding the ginger. Squeeze in lemon juice to taste.

Ginger Apple Fizz

"An apple a day" plus some ginger make this a fantastic cold-prevention juice.

- ½-inch piece ginger
- 1 pear
- 2 apples
- 2 ounces seltzer water

Process the ginger in a juicer, then the pear and apples. Add the seltzer to the juice, and stir well to combine.

The Dish on Ginger

The Good: Ginger is great for stomach problems and preventing and curing colds. It has anti-inflammatory properties that make it great for arthritis as well as preventing diseases related to chronic inflammation. The gingerol in it has actually been proven to cause cell death in ovarian cancer cells.

The Bad: Ginger has a powerful, distinctive "hot" flavor that many people don't care for. It can also be difficult to cut.

Green Carrot

You may want to add ¼ cup water to cut the strength of this juice. It's also really good if you add a jalapeño pepper.

- 2 cups spinach
- 1 head broccoli
- 6 Brussels sprouts
- 6 carrots

Process the spinach, broccoli, and Brussels sprouts in a juicer, then the carrots. Stir well to combine.

(28)

SEE YOUR WAY CLEAR— JUICING FOR HEALTHY EYES

Just like the rest of your body, your eyes need nutrients to function properly and stay healthy. Sadly, more than half of Americans over the age of sixty have some sort of vision loss caused by such diseases as cataracts and macular degeneration. On the positive side of these depressingly high numbers, there's plenty that you can do to keep from becoming an unfortunate statistic. By making some relatively simple, tasty additions to your diet, you can keep your eyes in tip-top shape and your vision good well into your dotage.

Vitamin A

There are six essential vitamins, minerals, and nutrients that work together to keep your eyes healthy. The first has been touted by that lovable, gray, carrot-toting rabbit Bugs Bunny for decades. That's right: carrots really do help your eyesight, at least in that they help keep your eyes healthy. The carotenoids and retinol (both forms of vitamin A) found in such produce as carrots, broccoli, spinach, and other orange and green fruits and veggies protect your eyes from free radicals.

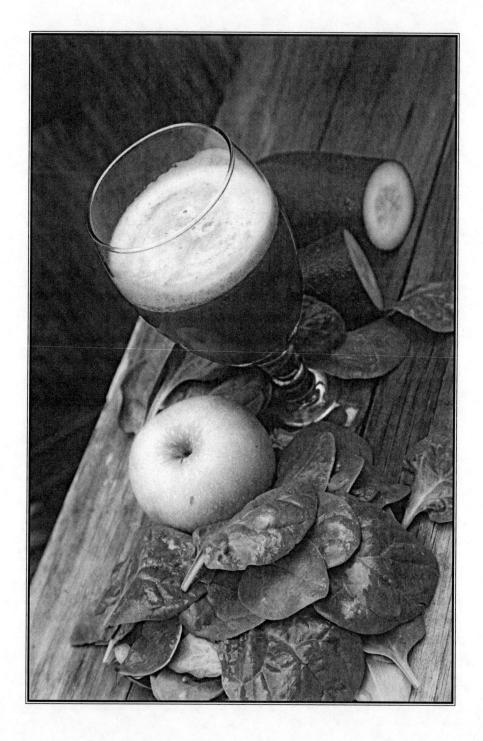

Zinc

Found in pumpkin seeds, tomatoes, and Napa cabbage, among others, zinc maintains your eyes by assisting with enzyme function in your retina. It's better to eat your zinc than to take it as a supplement because it can mess with the absorption of other nutrients.

Vitamin B Complex

Though each one benefits your eyes in a different way, the B vitamins are all necessary for good eye health. Riboflavin and niacin help keep your retinas healthy and B12 keeps your eyes lubricated. Look to leafy greens as well as citrus for some fantastic sources of B vitamins.

Vitamins C and E

Both of these antioxidants battle the free radicals responsible for degenerative eye disease. For vitamin C, look to dark green vegetables such as broccoli, bell peppers, and Brussels sprouts. Citrus fruits and kiwi are also good sources. For vitamin E, incorporate berries and green leafy veggies.

Now that you know what to look for, let's move on to the recipes that will provide you with everything you need to keep those eagle eyes!

All of the following recipes yield about two cups of juice.

Orange Carrot

Basic yet effective, this bright orange beverage will have you seeing (and looking) better for years to come.

- 1 yellow beet
- 6 carrots

- 1 orange

Process the beet and carrots in a juicer, then the orange. Stir well to combine.

Bugs's Juice

Follow in Bugs Bunny's footsteps and kick back those carrots. The addition of watercress here gives this juice a pleasantly peppery flavor.

- 1 bunch watercress
- 1 cup spinach
- 1 head broccoli

- 1 squash
- 5 carrots

Process the watercress, spinach, and broccoli in a juicer, then the squash and carrots. Stir well to combine.

C to See Juice

Note that some strict juice diets won't permit cantaloupe because of the amount of pulp that leaks through, but it's really good for you.

- 2 sweet potatoes
- 2 carrots

- 1 squash
- 1 cup cantaloupe

Process the sweet potatoes and carrots in a juicer, then the squash and cantaloupe. Stir well to combine.

The Dish on Cantaloupe

The Good: *Cantaloupe contains significant amounts of beta-carotene and vitamin A, two of the components necessary for eye health. It also contains other antioxidants that help protect your eyes from free-radical damage and diseases such as macular degeneration.*

The Bad: *Cantaloupe contains significant amounts of sugar and also tends to leak a large portion of its pulp into the juice.*

Nice to C You Juice

This juice will open your eyes in all kinds of ways. You may want to add some water to cut the strength of this a bit.

- 6 kale leaves
- 1 head broccoli
- 1 cup spinach
- 2 green bell peppers
- 4 carrots

Process the kale, broccoli, and spinach in a juicer, then the bell peppers and carrots. Stir well to combine.

Pumpkin Juice

This is a great way to bring a comforting taste of fall into your glass while also improving your health. You may enjoy adding some cinnamon to this juice as well.

- 6 carrots
- 2 sweet potatoes
- 2 squash
- 1 cup diced pumpkin

Process the carrots and sweet potatoes in a juicer, then the squash and pumpkin. Stir well to combine.

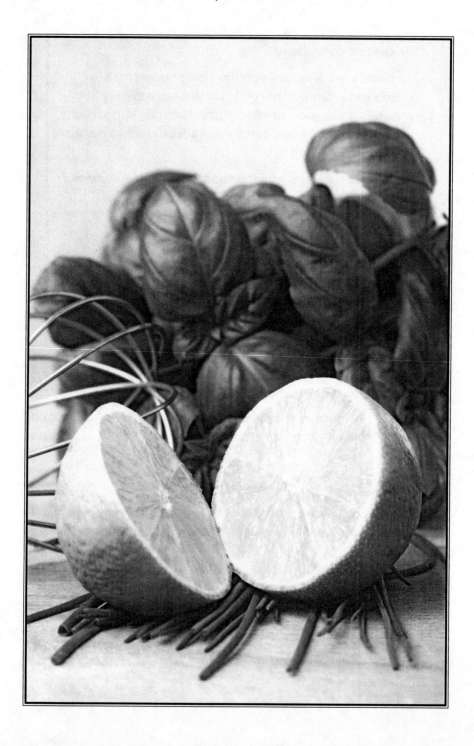

Sweet Potato Pie

This juice is nutritious as it is delicious. It really does taste like sweet potato pie! This will be a definite favorite if you enjoy its namesake.

- 4 sweet potatoes
- 4 carrots
- ½ teaspoon ground cinnamon
- ¼ teaspoon ground cloves

Process the sweet potatoes and carrots in a juicer. Add the cinnamon and cloves to the juice, and stir well to combine.

Veggie Boost

This juice is great for all manner of ailments. If you'd like extra spice, add some black pepper or even a jalapeño.

- 2 cups spinach
- 3 basil leaves
- 6 Brussels sprouts
- 1 fennel bulb
- 1 cucumber

Process the spinach, basil, and Brussels sprouts in a juicer, then the fennel and cucumber. Stir well to combine.

The Dish on Basil

The Good: *Packed with vitamin A, basil is great for your eyes and pleasing to your palate.*

The Bad: *Basil has a strong flavor and some people complain that it causes nausea when it's fresh, so use sparingly until you get used to it.*

Seeing Green

This one's pretty simple: it's green and great for your eyes!

- 2 cups spinach
- 1 head broccoli
- 1 cucumber

Process the spinach and broccoli in a juicer, then the cucumber. Stir well to combine.

Apriloupe Delight

A delightful, subtly sweet juice that will perk you up. You may enjoy some ginger in this as well.

- 3 carrots
- 2 apricots
- 1 cup diced cantaloupe

Process the carrots in a juicer, then the apricots and cantaloupe. Stir well to combine.

Green Popeye Juice

Make your eyes and body strong with this concoction. Feel free to throw a jalapeño in there for a kick if you'd like.

- 2 cups spinach
- 3 green bell peppers
- 4 celery stalks
- 1 cucumber

Process the spinach in a juicer, then the bell peppers, celery, and cucumber. Stir well to combine.

CONCLUSION

Juice fasting and cleansing has long been a concept incorporated by both the wise and the health conscious. Recently it has gained significant attention because of being adopted by celebrities as a way to lose weight and stay healthy. People use juice fasts as a way to cleanse their bodies and their minds.

Juicing Basics

Though the typical juice fast lasts from three to five days, there are as many different ways to juice as there are fruits and veggies to use. Some people opt to regularly drink only juice one day per week to give their systems a break from solid food, while others may fast for a month or longer. If you choose to do the latter, make sure that you speak to your health care professional and you're aware of all of the risks before you start—any extreme change in diet can cause significant side effects and even illness.

Though there's no doubt that fresh juice is good for you, there are definitely some pros and cons to participating in a fast. For instance, you're going to be depriving yourself of foods that you enjoy, and it can be a bit inconvenient to make juice to bring for lunch at work. On the other side of the coin, however, you're going to feel revitalized after a fast, and your system is going to get a good cleansing.

Juicing is a great way to get a flood of nutrients into your body so that it can flush out toxins and heal itself, but fasting isn't for everybody.

Because your body won't have to pull the nutrients from the fiber that they are generally encased in, you get a much more pure rush of nutrients, including sugars. If you're diabetic, this can be extremely harmful. There are other people for whom juicing may not be appropriate, so check with your doctor just to make sure that you're good to go.

Choosing a Juicer

One of the biggest decisions that you'll be making is what kind of juicer to buy. There are many different types, but they all operate in one of three ways. All of the other differences have to do with features, power, appearance, size, and price.

There really is no right or wrong juicer, because each one is designed with specific juicing needs in mind, so long as the one you choose is built to last. Some are designed for people who just want a glass of fresh orange juice every morning. Others are best for extracting the water content from grasses, such as wheatgrass and lemongrass. Some are great all-purpose machines that can handle the vast majority of fruits and vegetables, and some juicers can even do it all. The important thing to keep in mind is that your juicer should reflect your specific needs.

Make sure that your juicer has a good warranty, has enough power to meet your needs, is the right size for the job, and isn't difficult to use. As long as you are happy with its performance and are motivated to use it, that's all that matters. Talk to people, look around, read reviews, and comparison shop. Take your time and do it right, and you won't be disappointed!

So Cleanse Already!

Before you actually start your juice fast, there are some things that you need to do to prepare your body. It is, after all, a traumatic shock to your system. Not only are you going to be refraining from eating all solid foods, you're also going to be kicking all of your bad habits to the curb for the duration of the fast. This includes drinking alcohol, smoking cigarettes, downing caffeinated beverages, and other fun-but-destructive hobbies. You'll want to wean yourself off these things a little at a time, otherwise the first few days of your fast will be miserable.

In addition to kicking your bad habits slowly, you're going to want to start adding fresh juice to your diet so that your body has a chance to adjust. If you already drink fresh juice, then this isn't such a big deal, but if you don't, it really is smart to start incorporating juices a few days before you plan to exist on them alone!

When it comes to choosing your juices, try to stick with mostly vegetable juices. There are a couple of reasons for this. First of all, fruit juices contain much more sugar than vegetables do. This isn't necessarily a terrible thing from a caloric perspective, but it is from a digestive one when you're participating in a fast.

When you drink fruit juice, your body is absorbing that glucose and converting it immediately to sugar. This means that you're going to get a major energy pop. Plus, veggies tend to have more nutrients packed into them. Whether discussing fruits or veggies, there are those that stand out from the crowd nutritionally, which make them even more beneficial for juicing. Incorporate as many of those superstars as you possibly can.

There are also herbs and spices that add a significant nutritional and flavor boost to your juices, so don't forget to grab those while you're shopping for your produce, too.

What Are Your Juicing Goals?

The kind of juice fast that you do is ultimately dependent upon your goals. If you're feeling depressed, lethargic, and blah, it could be that you need a good detox. This is the primary reason that many people juice, and there are a ton of great juices out there to help you get your insides clean and healthy again.

If you're looking to juice in order to treat a particular illness or condition, such as arthritis, a cold, kidney stones, or even for weight loss, I've got you covered there as well.

Throughout this book, I've worked hard to pull together all of the facets of juicing that you need to know in order to complete your first fasting experience successfully. I've also included numerous tips and advice from folks who have already been there so that there are a few less bumps on your road to excellent health.

Happy juicing!